LOVE TRUMPS FEAR

About the Author

Patty Morell Bilhartz, MD, MPH, is licensed as an M.D. in the states of California and Texas, and works in a busy clinic in Northern California. She is board-certified by the American College of Preventive Medicine, with a specialty in Occupational Medicine. Dr. Bilhartz graduated from Texas A&M Medical School, completed an Internship in Internal Medicine at Scott & White Hospital in Temple, TX, and a specialty residency in Preventive Medicine, Public Health, and Environmental and Occupational Medicine at the University of Texas at Tyler Health Science Center.

She also holds a Master's Degree in Public Health from the Texas A&M Health Science Center School of Public Health, and a Certificate in "Botanicals and Health" from the University of Arizona Program in Integrative Medicine. She has done extensive study on preventive health, including specialty areas in lifestyle changes and hormone replacement therapy.

Dr. Bilhartz is a member of the Gold Humanism Honor Society, the Physicians Committee for Responsible Medicine, and the American College of Occupational and Environmental Medicine.

Before Dr. Bilhartz became a physician, she was a music teacher, and obtained a Master of Arts degree in music from Sam Houston State University. Dr. Bilhartz enjoys reading, gardening, and practicing yoga in her spare time. She and her husband, Terry, find great satisfaction in spending time with their children and grandchildren, and taking long walks in nature.

LOVE TRUMPS FEAR

8 Medical Insights to Heal Your Heart and Transform Your Health

Patty Morell Bilhartz, MD, MPH

2014
GREEN PUBLISHING HOUSE, LLC
College Station, Texas

Dedication

To my parents, Ann and Paul Morell, who lovingly gave of their lives to me so that I could learn to live and love;

To my children and grandchildren, Rocky, Lindsey, Preston, and Peyton Bilhartz and Teri, Scott, and Carson Maxwell who have responded to my ocean waves of love for them with even greater waves;

And to my husband Terry Bilhartz, my companion and soulmate on this life's journey, who has loved me throughout the wonderfully full serendipity of life that we have shared together now for over four decades;

How great the Divine is, and how grateful I am.

—Patty Ann Morell "Nani" Bilhartz

Table of Contents

INTRODUCTION:

East Meets West

I have talked about wanting to write a book for years, but have never done it. My excuses for not putting the pen to paper—or fingers to the computer keyboard—are much like others who think or say that they want to write a book, but never get around to it: not enough time, procrastination when there is time, lack of passion about the chosen subject, too far down on my priority list, etc. So, the book remained unwritten for far too long. However, a recent stunning, unexpected, life-changing circumstance presented me with both the time and passion that I needed to write this book, whose title is likely somewhat different than previous books' titles that I might have written before my catapulting life-experience. But, more about that later.

Authors say that we write about what we need most to learn, and this book is no exception. The words on the pages of this book come from deep within my heart and soul and are written to you, a fellow sojourner along the path that we call "life." My desire is that the insights that I share with you would resonate within your heart and bring to you optimal health and a blessed future, no matter what your current circumstances or health status might be.

As a medical doctor (M.D.) trained in the United States, over the years I have become very curious about and furthered my knowledge of other medical philosophies and approaches including osteopathic, homeopathic, chiropractic, acupuncture, Ayurvedic, herbal, Chinese, energy, mind-body, alternative, holistic, preventive, functional, and integrative medicine. I have discovered in my practice that when I study about and then become open to implementing a variety of healing approaches for my patients, they seem to benefit the most. Even if there appears to be no immediate cure for the physical condition with which my patient presents, I find that some form of healing in the mind, body, or soul always can occur when the patient and I work compassionately in tandem.

One aspect of medicine that I find particularly interesting relates to the study of energy and how it presents itself in our bodies via electrical conduction and energy meridians. Although western medicine recognizes and even measures the ability of our hearts and brains to conduct electricity, which is a form of energy, discussions of the presence of energy centers and meridians in our bodies traditionally have been more compatible with eastern than western philosophies.

Energy meridians stem from the eastern understanding that our human bodies have seven major energy centers from and along which our body energy flows. These energy centers begin at the base of our spines and move up our bodies to the crown of our heads. Energy medicine teaches that if any of our centers are weak or out of balance, the energy flow of our bodies becomes blocked, and our bodies can detour from optimal health.

Our energy centers become weakened and blocked when we allow life's fearful stimuli to diminish our innate love: love for ourselves and others. Fear begins to trump love when our lifestyles become hurried, stressed, filled with suboptimal food, and devoid of body movement. Balancing our hormones, establishing clarity of mind, implementing truth and forgiveness, following Divine inner guidance, and loving ourselves and others enough to follow abundant and compassionate lifestyles, all these can lead us back to our highest nature where we discover that we can live our lives with the truth that love trumps fear, rather than the other way around.

I have chosen to organize this book around our seven energy centers—sometimes referred to as our energy chakras—as we discuss medical insights from both the east and the west that can assist our bodies in keeping the seven centers strong, balanced, and free flowing. As we discover ways to live in the flow of optimal energy, my hope is that your heart will find healing and your health will be transformed.

"Chapter 1: Safety and Security: Recognizing I Am Enough" digs deep into our root energy center or first chakra at the base of our spine that stems from safety and security. Each of us has experiences from

childhood and adulthood that we have allowed to wound us and make us feel insecure and less whole. These wounds can take their toll on our health and relationships if not loved into oblivion. Becoming aware of our inner beauty brings us into new levels of wholeness and health.

"Chapter 2: Pleasure: Experiencing Balanced Hormones" examines our second energy center, or chakra of pleasure located in our lower abdominal area, which is organized by our hormones and neurotransmitters in our physical bodies, as well as our thoughts felt and expressed. Imbalanced hormones and neurotransmitters can wreak havoc with our health, and often just a little tweaking can make a world of difference in how we feel and view the world.

"Chapter 3: Abundance: Embracing Compassionate Living" investigates our third energy center, or chakra spaced around the navel where abundance resides. Developing an awareness that all of our needs are met brings us into a world of plenty versus a world of lack. When we learn how to see the world as a playground rather than as a battleground, and the glass as half-full versus half-empty, we offer ourselves gifts of abundant living.

As we exercise the generous autonomy that we have been given in many of our lifestyle choices, including **Fabulous Food, Fantastic Fitness,** and **Festive Fun,** we begin to see that genetics plays a very small role in our health compared to our wise choices of conscious living.

"Chapter 4: Love: Outshining the Shadows of Depression and Anxiety" develops our fourth energy chakra of lovingkindness that finds its resting place in our heart. Practicing daily lovingkindness both for ourselves and for others, along with educating ourselves toward nurturing thoughts and lifestyle behaviors, can assist us in moving out of the shadows of depression and anxiety into the light of hope and love. Medications also may be beneficial in the short- and/or long-term as we continue to cultivate practices of compassionate living.

"Chapter 5: Truth and Forgiveness: Making Peace with Chronic Pain and Illness" moves us into our fifth energy center of truth and forgiveness located in our throat, where we can gain the transformational tools to overcome chronic pain and illness. Once we can accept the truth about any situation and begin the process of forgiveness for ourselves and others, we achieve the freedom that sets into motion the

healing of our physical, mental, and emotional selves. We will discuss practical medical tools to reduce pain and increase our ability to live life as victors instead of victims.

"Chapter 6: Clarity: Choosing Nurturing Thoughts" looks into our sixth chakra located between the eyebrows which represents clarity of mind. This is our "third eye," where we empower ourselves through inspirational thoughts that can support our process of healing to wholeness. We experience creativity and joy when we learn how to choose nurturing thoughts through conscious practice. And, our health responds in miraculous ways.

"Chapter 7: Guidance: Finding Your Center" culminates with our seventh chakra of guidance, strategically placed at the top of our head. The energy resonating from this center assists us in making wise decisions about our health and wellness. As we learn ways through meditation and devotional practices to remain centered in our highest selves of lovingkindness, we experience a Divine Connection that results in an overflowing of beauty and love in our lives.

"Chapter 8: The Flow: Reframing the Impostors of Good Luck, Bad Luck" puts it all together by

reminding us that optimal health transpires when each energy center of the body works in tandem with the others to produce a harmonious chorus of unimpeded energy flow throughout the body. As we make conscious daily choices to move out of a fear-controlled life to a life based on lovingkindness, we begin to view all of life's events —whether they are perceived as good or bad by the world— as lessons to be learned and experiences that ultimately work together for our good. We glimpse the amazing life that we can have when we trust its serendipitous twists and turns and surrender to the flow of the moment, realizing that fear is an impostor that robs us of joy and happiness, and that love always trumps fear, because only love truly exists. Miraculously, our hearts are healed and our health is transformed as we become love to ourselves and others.

"*Epilogue: Join Our Community*" gives us practical ways to connect with and support each other along our individual roads of healing. Our community offers love and acceptance to all, no matter where we are on our journey.

The book title promises 8 medical insights that have the capacity to heal our hearts and transform our health, one step at a time. When received and practiced, these insights can provide accurate and deep intuitive revelations that can gradually move us from fear to love, in every moment and in every circumstance. I invite you to get started in the healing process with me as we hobble, walk, run, jog, skip, leap, and dance our way through the full serendipity of life and love!

CHAPTER 1:

Safety and Security: Recognizing I Am Enough

I was four years old when I proudly but anxiously remember going to the Julia Private School for aptitude testing. My parents staunchly believed that I was ready to begin first grade; however, the school administrators naturally had some misgivings about a four year old attending their school as a first grader. The tests were offered as a compromise: if I performed well enough on them, the administrators would consider admitting me to their first grade class. The pre-placement tests lasted two days, and the only instructions that I recall being given from my parents were to "do my best." I did not want to disappoint them or the school administrators, so I gave the testing "my all" in the hopes that I would be seen as "smart enough" to enter first grade at Julia School.

My mother, a first grade teacher and speech therapist before my birth, tells me that I was so bored as a very young child that she began to teach me to read at the age of three. Apparently, I had a predilection for phonics and caught on to reading quickly, so that by the age of four, I was reading at a third grade level. My parents felt it would have been a travesty not to continue my education more formally, so they began to look for a school that would be open-minded enough to enroll me in a first grade class at the age of four. I must have done pretty well on the entrance exams for Julia School, because I began first grade soon after the testing took place, and thus embarked on an education that culminated in completion of high school at age 15 and college graduation two weeks after my twentieth birthday. (I later completed two Master's Degrees and graduated from Medical School at the age of 55, but that is fodder for another chapter.)

My father was a minister, and in the earlier days of his career, our family moved often, which meant at each new school that I was to attend, I underwent placement testing in order to convince the new administrators and teachers that I could handle schoolwork in a classroom that was two years beyond the grade of my chronological age. We moved to Texas in September when I was nine and in the sixth grade, and I distinctly remember that several of my classmates had already turned twelve because they had a fall birthday, and my birthday was not until late spring, which made the age gap even more apparent. Thus, I intensified my defense to "prove" to yet another group of educators and classmates that I was "smart enough" to compete with classmates that were significantly older than I. Fortunately, I was tall enough that I looked the part of my grade, although that made little difference to the Department of Motor Vehicles when issuing a Driver's License that my classmates obtained as sophomores in high school, but I did not receive until after high school completion.

Please understand that I am not complaining about the possibly truncated childhood that I experienced, nor do I feel that my parents made a mistake in attempting to challenge me intellectually by placing me in school at a young age. In fact, I am grateful to them for their love and devotion to me, always seeking the path for me that they felt was best. And, there were many benefits about being two years "ahead" in school. For one, my brain was challenged to learn and compete, and secondly, I developed a curiosity for learning that has served me well my entire life.

Despite these advantages, however, this quest for competitive learning gradually became rather addictive. The more that I equated my identity with my intelligence, the more my external self-esteem expanded. But as I learned over the years, self-esteem that is built from the outside in is tenuous at best, and must continuously be re-proven. The constant need to prove my aptitudes to myself and others became a ruthless taskmaster, and I learned quickly that I was only as good as my last test grade or precocious behavior.

I also believe that this emphasis on my external self contributed to my growing desire to engage in patterns and behaviors that would please others, and so I routinely denied myself immediate pleasures or self-expression in order to be the obedient child that I knew others wanted me to be. Although I am truly appreciative of my parents' diligence in advancing my education, I do feel that this need to constantly demonstrate to others that I was intellectually worthy of my grade placement set me up for a continual striving to achieve more and more and to be as perfect as possible. Over time, these behaviors and beliefs became cumbersome to continue and impossible to sustain without me feeling that I was disappointing others, but even more crucially, disappointing myself and God.

To illustrate, I remember that I took swimming lessons at the age of four, and at the end of a lesson, the instructor threw me out into what I thought was the deep water. I truly thought that I was drowning, and recall that my short life flashed before me. I quickly asked God to forgive me for anything wrong that I had ever done, and prayed that I would go to heaven. Shortly thereafter, the instructor plucked me out of the water, but the experience remains vivid in my memory. Even at age four, I was convinced that I was lacking.

The ancient Hawaiians tell a story about "The Bowl of Light," that illustrates how at birth we know that we are enough, but over time lose this innate knowledge and question everything about ourselves because we feel so inadequate.[1] This "Bowl of Light"—the pure container of light that each person possesses at birth—continuously fills and ultimately is covered up with rocks that represent times where we listened to others' advice over our own intuitive direction, where we "sold our souls" in attempts to make others pleased with our behaviors, and where we accepted what others said about us and then allowed those beliefs to shape our lives in inauthentic directions. As the story goes, over time, feelings of fear, anger, and worry cause more rocks to be dropped into the bowl, whereas attitudes of love, happiness, and trust allow the innate light to shine. If we accumulate enough rocks, then the light can no longer be seen because it is blocked by the rocks that now fill the bowl. The process of losing our shining light can be reversed by re-remembering our beautiful, innocent, unique self, and taking courageous steps to express it in the world in loving ways of service to others. As we remember that we are enough and travel with instead of against the flow of life, the rocks of fear and inauthenticity gradually drop out of our basket, and our innate light once again shines brightly.

In the same respect, a quote from the book *The Polar Express* by Chris Van Allsburg conveys this message of what happens when we question whether our innate calling is enough: "At one time, most of my friends could hear the bell, but as years passed, it fell silent for all of them. Even Sarah found one Christmas that she could no longer hear its sweet sound. Though I've grown old, the bell still rings for me, as it does for all who truly believe."[2]

I have shared with you my story, but I am sure that you have very similar stories where you felt your first chakra of safety and security that is represented by the base of the spine wrenched at its very root. You probably even knew at the time or realized later that you had "sold your true self for a bowl of porridge," as is so aptly conveyed in the Biblical story of Jacob and Esau. In this story, Jacob used trickery and a bowl of porridge to steal his first-born brother's familial birthright, while his brother Esau exchanged his more prized blessing for a simple meal.[3]

In short, we all possess a myriad of wounds that have accumulated from childhood that ache to be healed. How do we start this healing process? How can we fully embrace that we are enough, despite what anyone else said or did that wounded us in the past? How do we uncover our innate light and our conscious ability to hear the bell? Does love for ourselves truly have the ability to trump our fears?

Over the years in my medical practice, I have discussed with many patients that they are worth loving and taking care of themselves. Often, this means stopping smoking, losing weight, exercising more, removing themselves from toxic relationships, or getting needed sleep at night. These conversations occasionally produce excuses, but more often than not, these discussions result in tears and grateful appreciation for my willingness to take the time to encourage them to see themselves as lovable.

Western medical interventions rarely involve conversations from physicians to patients on the importance of seeing themselves as worthy of love and care. Likely this may be because addressing emotions and self-awareness are frequently relegated to the specialty of psychiatry, and often the patient is only referred to a mental health professional if the patient seems so unstable that the primary care physician or family member worries that the patient might harm him/herself or someone else. To complicate matters even further, love for oneself in the western world is often seen as conceit or arrogance, and thus is discouraged. In contrast, eastern medicine designates the first root chakra as the universal energy center from which self-worth and security emanate, and every person is encouraged to cultivate and deepen self-love in order to move toward optimal health.

If loving ourselves is such an essential component for both inner and outer health, how do we learn to release fear and accept love for ourselves, and in the process find that this self-love restores our health and actually frees us to love and serve others more fully? I believe that for each of us to love ourselves with enough passion and see ourselves as "Enough" involves awareness, acceptance, and practice.

Consider the following daily practices to begin transforming fear into love.

MEDICAL INSIGHT #1:
I AM ENOUGH

1. Set aside approximately thirty minutes where you will not be interrupted. Sit in a comfortable position and close your eyes.

   Transport your thoughts back to the time when you were in your mother's womb. Envision a radiating light surrounding you that carries within it peace and love. Imagine that your heart is opening up to let go of fear and embrace love.

   Now, gradually allow your thoughts to move through your life chronologically. Pause with any thought that produces emotion and let it go with love. Send forgiveness to others and to yourself as you let the thought go. Remind yourself as you let go that "I Am Enough."

   Continue this exercise of remembering and letting go with love as time allows. Provide yourself ample time to go through your life's emotional memories, even if it means doing this exercise of letting go repeatedly for as many sessions as you need. Make this practice a daily routine, where you take the time to open your heart and let go of any feelings of fear of not being enough. Allow love to wash over you as you acknowledge that "I Have Always Been Enough" and "I Am Enough." When you replace fear with love, the energy in your root chakra will flow without interruption, and your open heart will heal your body, mind, and emotions.

2. Look in a mirror multiple times daily, or whenever you are in the same room with a mirror. Gaze deeply into your eyes, and say, "I Am Enough!"

   Repeat this phrase while adding other complimentary phrases about yourself, such as, "I Love Me," "I Am Absolutely Amazing," and "I Am Complete Just As I Am." You will find how difficult and awkward it is initially to make such deep connections with yourself. You also will note how quickly you begin to find fault with yourself as you look into the mirror. Gently bring your thoughts and words back to kind and generous compliments toward yourself.

   The longer you practice this exercise, the easier it will become, and the more love that you will feel for yourself and for others. Louise Hay, the metaphysical writer and author, makes this practice of looking into the mirror daily a mainstay of her day, and finds that it has transformed her life and health as it has for many others that have begun this practice.[4] Give it a try!

As we learn to discard those aspects of ourselves that breed fear, and begin to cultivate loving ourselves unconditionally, we find that our heart begins to heal and our health is transformed.

CHAPTER 2:

Pleasure: Experiencing Balanced Hormones

I was 29 when I underwent a hysterectomy that included the removal of my uterus and one ovary. At the time, I didn't see any other viable alternative, since imaging showed that I had at least one tumor on my ovary and an enlarged uterus. More significantly to me, I had constant abdominal pain that made it uncomfortable for me to hold my two young children on my lap, and experienced irregular, heavy periods. I also had decided that I did not want any more children, and although my husband expressed some ambivalence about whether or not he wanted a third child, this surgery would answer that question decisively.

My surgeon told me that my one ovary that would be intact after the surgery would produce all the hormones that I needed, and thus I would feel well and not need to take any replacement hormones. However, this advice did not prove to be true for me, because after the surgery, my energy levels plummeted, I became very depressed, experienced daily hot flashes and night sweats, and within a few months, gained 30 pounds. I also gradually began experiencing new abdominal pain that felt very much like the old pain before my hysterectomy, and repeat imaging six months later showed that my remaining ovary now was encased with a large tumor.

Six months after my hysterectomy, I underwent another abdominal surgery to remove the tumor and what was left of the remaining ovary. I gladly accepted the oral estrogen that my physician offered me now that I had no ovaries, but my symptoms did not improve, even though my physician prescribed several different synthetic oral and injectable estrogen and progesterone formulations. After several months of continued symptoms, 20 more pounds gained, and two second opinions later, I saw a physician who said that I likely was not absorbing these forms of hormones, and he prescribed a bioidentical estrogen patch for me to use.

Almost overnight, my energy returned, my depression and hot flashes/night sweats resolved, and within a few months, I lost the weight that I had gained. My physician told me that I did not need progesterone since I had no uterus, and testosterone supplementation was never mentioned. I was not a physician at that time, knew very little about the major role that hormones played in overall health, and did not question what my doctor told me. I was just thankful that I felt better!

Several years later, I began doing research on the effects of early hysterectomies and treatment with bioidentical hormones, and discovered that controversy abounded in the field of hormone replacement therapy (HRT). I later went to medical school, and experienced first-hand that western physicians are taught very little about optimizing hormones in both males and females, other than replacing deficient hormones via the prescribing of a few synthetic drugs. No wonder I had such difficulty finding help!

Some of my research brought me to Dr. Uzzi Reiss's seminal book *Natural Hormone Balance for Women*, where I read clinical vignettes by an experienced treating physician that described the benefits of HRT.[1] Over the next several years, I sold my music business and went to medical school, reading just about everything available to me in both the popular media and in the scientific journals regarding hormone replacement therapy for both men and women. This included Dr. Christiane Northrup's amazing treatises on *The Wisdom of Menopause and Women's Bodies, Women's Wisdom*,[2,3] which combined both western and eastern medicinal approaches to optimizing hormones. By the time that I graduated from medical school, women's health had become my great interest, not only because it was an exciting and complex subject, but also because I had personally experienced the importance of properly functioning hormones for overall good health, and I wanted to help my patients with the knowledge that I had gained.

I have learned that hormones can be balanced in several ways, and each complements the other. Hormone replacement therapies and supplements as needed, together with lifestyle changes (discussed in more detail in subsequent chapters), can assist in optimizing hormone levels. However, we can't stop there. Because the second chakra circles around the reproductive centers that represent pleasure areas of our body, the thoughts that we think provide the energy in these areas that also can help to determine how much pleasure we feel. This chapter will focus on the physical aspects of hormone balancing, and a discussion of the mental or mind-body connection of the power that our thoughts play in controlling our pleasure centers will be offered in Chapter 6.

Our body touts a myriad of hormones, but in this chapter, we are going to examine three of the steroid hormones—the sex hormones estrogen, testosterone, and progesterone (whether or not a woman has a uterus) in women, and testosterone in men—and the parts they play, in the overall health of our bodies. When our sex hormones are balanced, our pleasure centers are normalized, our weight and moods stabilize, and our brain functions well. Let's first look at some of the symptoms that imbalanced hormones can produce, and then we will examine how to optimize our hormone levels through a variety of ways.

Symptoms of imbalanced hormones fall into three categories that I call the 3 F's: "Fat, Frazzled, and Foggy." When our hormones are imbalanced, we can experience out-of-control food cravings that can lead to excessive weight gain; we can feel edgy, anxious, depressed, compulsive, uninterested in sex, and on an emotional roller coaster; we can describe "brain fog" that is often defined by relentless fatigue and difficulty in focusing, remembering, and sleeping. Causes of imbalanced hormones are complex and can result in part from aging, genetic predisposition, and environmental toxins, but often stem predominantly from chronic elevation of another steroid hormone, cortisol, which is known to be one of the hormones that our body releases when it senses a stressful situation.

Cortisol is meant to be at its highest levels early in the day, and then is supposed to gradually decrease as the day goes on and we prepare for sleep. However, because we often perceive our lives to be chronically stressful, cortisol levels may stay continuously elevated, and thus other hormones that are not considered essential to keeping us alive respond by remaining at very low levels. Specifically, when cortisol is high, estrogen, progesterone, and testosterone stay low, and low levels of any of these hormones can contribute to symptoms of the 3 F's. Think about it like this: if you found yourself in the middle of a terrorist attack, you would not think about eating, sleeping, or having sex; instead, your heart would be beating rapidly in order to increase the blood flow to your body so that you would be able to run quickly from danger.

If you suspect that you might have non-optimal levels of these sex hormones based on the presence of some of the above symptoms, you may wish to have your levels checked through blood, saliva or urine testing, depending on your physician's preference. You also can request to have other steroid hormones tested, such as DHEAs and cortisol. Although you may ask your physician to check your hormone levels, you often will find that western-trained physicians may be reluctant to do this. You may even find that your physician will minimize your symptoms by saying that they are "common," or present just because you are "getting older." If so, you might consider working with a functional or integrative medicine physician who has been trained and has more experience in managing imbalanced hormones.

If your hormone testing shows that your hormones are not at optimal levels, then you can discuss with your physician or healthcare practitioner the options you have to assist you in regaining hormonal balance, and whether or not you might be a candidate for HRT. Although there have been conflicting past study results regarding the safety of HRT, it has become clearer over the last several years that for most women and men, balancing hormone levels actually decreases our risks for developing many chronic diseases, including cardiovascular disease, certain cancers, osteoporosis, and dementia.[4,5,6,7,8,9]

Two types of HRT are available: synthetic and bioidentical. Synthetic hormones are generated in a lab, and are slightly different chemically from the endogenous hormones that our bodies produce. Bioidentical hormones are created in a laboratory as well, but their molecular structures mimic the molecular structures of the hormones that the body produces, which potentially increases the likelihood that they will be better accepted and more appropriately put to use by the body. A number of recent studies show that bioidentical hormones may have a better safety profile as well.[10,11] Bioidentical HRT is available as a prescription in a pill, cream, gel, spray, patch, or pellet form, and, depending on the medication, can be obtained at a regular pharmacy or at a compounding pharmacy where the hormone is compounded for each patient per the physician's prescription.

Many supplements have been shown to support hormone balancing. Some of the most important from my perspective include Vitamin D, Vitamin B complex, probiotics, omega-3 fatty acids, and melatonin. We will discuss in the next chapter the importance of Vitamin D in regulating every cell in the body. B complex assists with energy levels and optimal neurological function. Probiotics regulate the microbiome of healthy bacteria in the gut that contributes to overall digestive and immunological health. Omega-3 fatty acids are beneficial for the heart, brain, skin, and most body systems, including the reproductive and neurological systems. Melatonin is a hormonal supplement that can be purchased over the counter, and can be a helpful sleep aid.

Supplemental herbs also can be beneficial. Rhodiola can decrease symptoms of depression, fatigue, and lack of focus, while Valerian and Passion Flower can improve sleep and also reduce anxiety.[12,13]

If you decide with your practitioner that supplements and/or herbs might be beneficial, you will want to purchase them from a company that produces "nutraceutical grade" supplements – supplements that have undergone a rigorous process of quality control to ensure that they are in a bioavailable form that is readily usable by the body, free from harmful substances and contaminants, and that the dose stated on the package is accurate.

Lifestyle changes that will reduce your symptoms include daily exercise, compassionate living, healthy food and thought choices, and stress reduction. These will be discussed in future chapters.

Our sex hormones, when balanced, bring us physical pleasure that can extend well into our golden years, as well as mental and emotional stability. When our hearts are emotionally whole, our brains are mentally stable, and our bodies feel good, we bring a unique beauty to the world around us as we serve ourselves and others. It is not surprising that our second energy chakra centers around pleasure, because as we discover pleasure and contentment for ourselves, we are then better able to help others to find the same.

Consider the following to assist in balancing your hormones.

MEDICAL INSIGHT #2: BALANCING YOUR HORMONES

1. Educate yourself on the importance of hormonal balancing and the best ways to go about it.

   Select one or two books from this list of recommended books to start your learning process:

   Dr. Christiane Northrup's *The Wisdom of Menopause*[2] and *Women's Bodies, Women's Wisdom;*[3]

   Dr. Sara Gottfried, *The Hormone Cure;*[14]

   Dr. Lissa Rankin, *Mind Over Medicine;*[15]

Dr. Uzzi Reiss, *Natural Hormone Balance;*[1]

Dr. Erika Schwartz, *The Hormone Solution;*[16]

Dr. Abraham Morgentaler, *Testosterone For Life;*[17]

and Dr. Robert S. Tan, *The Andropause Mystery.*[18]

2. Find a physician or healthcare practitioner whom you trust and who shares your philosophy of wellness and desire to bring your hormones to their optimal balance.

You may feel comfortable working with your current physician or healthcare practitioner; however, if you find him/her resistant to working with you in the area of hormonal balancing, you can seek a specialist in holistic, functional, or integrative medicine. One way to start would be to contact a local compounding pharmacy and ask for a recommendation for a local holistic, functional, or integrative physician/ practitioner. Other websites that provide directories of physicians/practitioners that might be helpful include:

International College of Integrative Medicine: http://www.icimed.com/index.php

American Board of Integrative Holistic Medicine: http://www.abihm.org/search-doctors

Arizona Center for Integrative Medicine: http://integrativemedicine.arizona.edu/alumni.html

The Institute for Functional Medicine:
http://www.functionalmedicine.org/practitioner_search.aspx?id=117

The American Academy of Anti-Aging Medicine:
http://www.a4m.com/directory.html

3. If you have difficulty finding a suitable practitioner in your area, consider testing with an independent lab that can then refer you to a practitioner for follow-up.

   Three reputable labs that provide hormonal testing are www.canaryclub.org, www.lifeextension.com, and www.precisionhormones.com.

4. Follow your practitioner's advice regarding HRT and supplements as needed. Make certain that you work with your practitioner to buy nutraceutical grade supplements as previously discussed in this chapter.

   Two websites that can help you to determine appropriate quality supplements are www.consumerlab.com and www.usp.org.

5. Remember the importance of the mind-body connection in stabilizing your hormone levels.

   Engage in daily lifestyle choices that include physical and mental exercise, compassionate living, healthy food and thought choices, and stress reduction. We will further discuss the mind-body connection and healthy lifestyle choices in upcoming chapters.

As we enter into a plan to balance our hormones, we will find that our emotional heart will heal and our health will be transformed. Then, it becomes easier for us to discover ways daily to replace fear with love.

CHAPTER 3:

Abundance: Embracing Compassionate Living

Although in my early adulthood I always tried to eat "healthy" and provide my body with daily exercise, I really began to get more serious about a lifestyle of "compassionate living" shortly before my 40th birthday, when I was given a life-altering diagnosis of myasthenia gravis.

Myasthenia gravis is a rare autoimmune neuromuscular disease that causes muscles to fatigue with repetitive use. At the time of my diagnosis, I had been a pianist and music teacher for over 2 decades. About a year before my diagnosis, I noticed that I had begun to have some subtle clumsiness when playing the piano or writing with a pen. Over the next few months, I developed increasingly noticeable weakness in my legs after repetitive use, and I felt that I had become more forgetful than normal. I was concerned that I might have a brain tumor, but initial medical testing did not show any abnormalities, so I continued to work until one day while I was sitting on the floor teaching a music class of young children, my legs became so weak that I could not get off the floor. I literally had to crawl to the phone to call for assistance.

After another month or so of additional testing, including an inaccurate diagnosis of amyotrophic lateral sclerosis (Lou Gehrig's disease)—known to be a virtual death sentence within a few years after diagnosis—I was given the diagnosis of myasthenia gravis. Within a month, I traveled with my husband to New York City to undergo a surgical procedure called a thymectomy, where my thymus gland was removed in an attempt to slow down and perhaps even halt my body's autoimmune response that was keeping my muscles fatigued with use. The thymectomy was successful, and after several months of being in and out of a wheelchair, I found myself regaining my strength and re-entering the world again as a relatively "normal" 40 year old.

Although myasthenia gravis is rarely fatal, the life-changing experience of coming to grips with my mortality and facing possible permanent disability propelled me to make changes to my current lifestyle habits. I focused more on slowing down and living in the moment and less on fighting the minor irritations of life, and I made more time to sleep and take better care of myself. Taking "better care of myself" included eating less sugar and more vegetables, walking mindfully—which was my favorite form of exercise—and engaging in a daily devotional and exercise practice that helped to minimize stress, maximize body strength, and connect me with a higher spiritual power.

Over the next decade, I began to seek what it was that I truly wanted to do with my life. My myasthenia was asymptomatic most of the time, and I had heard a renowned physician say that if a woman made it to the age of 50 without developing a chronic disease of diabetes, cancer, or heart disease, she would likely live into her nineties. (Likewise, a non-smoking male who makes it to the age of 45 without developing diabetes, high blood pressure, or high cholesterol has only a 1.4% chance of developing a cardiovascular event in his lifetime. Unfortunately, only 5% of all males fall into this category.[1]) The thought that I fell into the category of likely living into my nineties based on my lack of the above chronic diseases, and thus might be just completing the first half of my life, and the fact that women in my family lived long, healthy lives fueled me to seriously consider a career change.

I had married at a young age, and the first few years of our marriage, we moved several times while my husband was completing two graduate degrees and getting started in his career. I assisted him in achieving his goals by supporting us as a medical secretary and completing my undergraduate degree as time allowed. I ended up choosing to obtain a graduate degree and pursue a career in music rather than medicine or science, even though I had obtained an undergraduate degree in biology, partly because our frequent moves precluded me from being in one place long enough to complete any medical training, and partly because I ultimately decided that a music career would allow me to teach part-time from my home while I was raising my children.

However, although I enjoyed teaching music and ultimately extended my home teaching into a full-time career where I owned my own music business, I continued to maintain an interest in medicine. Once our kids were grown and the call of medicine's voice began to overpower my passion for music teaching, I decided to return to school with the possible goal of completing the necessary medical prerequisites that would allow me to apply to medical school. Beginning that road at age 47 was not easy, but ended up being worth it, as I was accepted to medical school at age 50.

I believe that the grace of the Divine and my continued healthy lifestyle of eating well and exercising daily, along with getting enough sleep and minimizing stress, allowed me to successfully complete my medical training at age 59. Over my twelve years of prerequisite study and medical training, my healthy eating evolved from eating less sugar and more vegetables and exercising daily, to what I now would describe as an abundant lifestyle of "compassionate living."

I had never eaten a lot of meat, particularly red meat, but by the time that I entered medical school in 2005, the only meat that I was eating was fish, and then over the next two years, as I began to read and study more about compassionate living, I gradually stopped eating fish. Moving from choosing to eat less meat for the sake of being healthy to choosing not to eat meat out of sensitivity for the treatment of animals propelled me into a new world of compassionate living—a spectacularly abundant and conscious world that continues to bring me great inner peace as well as the by-products of the rewards of healthy living.

It is interesting that our third chakra centers around the solar plexus—the energy center in the body just below the navel—and includes the liver and digestive system. Without the energy from this center, we cannot move out of inertia into action. The third chakra harnesses a combination of will and power to help us achieve our goals. When these two words are combined, we have the word "willpower." Unfortunately, this word often takes on a pejorative context when it comes to diet or exercise, because we frequently can feel that we have no "willpower" when it comes to making and sustaining healthy choices.

Our third chakra also represents abundance and that we can trust that all our needs are met. Viewing the world from an abundance mentality verses a mentality of lack brings us into alignment with our inner wisdom. Furthermore, the center of our deep inner wisdom—sometimes called our intuition—is often represented by our gut. How many times have you heard someone refer to a "gut feeling" that he or she had but did not listen to, and suffered negative consequences as a result? So, when we put all of this together, if we allow our inner wisdom to lead us to wise choices that encompass compassionate living, we will find that this lifestyle of healthy choices does not bring us into scarcity, but brings us into abundance. Let's examine compassionate living under the lens of abundance, and see how this shift can make a difference in the choices that we make, and the feelings that result.

I think that what makes me so enthusiastic about compassionate living—including healthy eating, regular exercise, and daily attention to stress reduction and spiritual growth—is that it is more than just a diet, exercise, or stress reduction plan. Compassionate living is an abundant way of treating ourselves lavishly with great lovingkindness, approval, and respect. It is a way of saying, "I am worth loving." It is a way of discarding all of the baggage of fear that surrounds diet, exercise, and stress, and replacing it with love for ourselves and all earthly creatures. And, when we daily practice and implement a compassionate lifestyle, the bonus of amazing physical and psychological benefits follow.

What are some of these benefits that result from engaging in a lifestyle of compassionate living? In addition to the advantages of maintaining a healthy weight, having more energy, and lowering body inflammation and pain, many major chronic diseases can be avoided when we implement a compassionate lifestyle. How is this possible? In the past, geneticists taught us that our genes predetermine and control our health, so we believed that chronic diseases such as diabetes and heart disease and even many cancers, if they existed in our close family members, likely would develop in us as well. Scientist Dr. Bruce Lipton in his book *The Biology of Belief* introduces us to the new concept of epigenetics that removes much of the powerlessness that we previously thought existed when thinking about our genes. The principle of epigenetics demonstrates that although we may have a genetic propensity for diabetes, for example, these genes likely will need to be "turned on" in order for the diabetes to be expressed in our body. It appears that our thoughts and lifestyle behaviors can actively control and even turn on or off many of our genes. Thus, by engaging in nurturing thoughts and compassionate lifestyles, we literally can turn on many healthful genes and almost certainly prevent many unhealthful genes from being activated.[2]

I was stunned when I read that upwards of 90% of Type 2 diabetes (the type that generally develops in adulthood), 80% of cardiovascular disease, and 60% of cancer are virtually preventable with a lifestyle of compassionate living.[3] These statistics help to raise our awareness that many of our health outcomes are under our control, and we can embrace the truth that often we are in the driver's seat and not mere passengers as we travel on life's road.

I like to describe compassionate living by dividing it into 3 categories: **Fabulous Food**, **Fantastic Fitness**, and **Festive Fun**. **Fabulous Food** includes eating a colorful plant-based diet; **Fantastic Fitness** encompasses regularly moving our bodies in enjoyable ways; and **Festive Fun** promotes living in the moment, laughing more, reducing stress, emphasizing spiritual growth, and treating ourselves to a cessation of addictive habits such as smoking and substance use. Let's now consider each of the three areas in more depth.

Choosing **Fabulous Food** does not have to be punitive or a denial of pleasure; in fact, choosing **Fabulous Food** can be abundant living at its best! Plant-based choices that emphasize meals centered around veggies instead of meat, and include a plate full of rainbow colors of fruits and vegetables and small amounts of protein sources such as legumes, nuts, soy, gluten-free grains, and nondairy milks/ cheeses can be delightfully delicious. Meals focused on veggies are full of fiber, which helps to keep sugar levels stable and satiation levels high, and promotes healthy elimination. If you think that you don't like most veggies, start with one or two veggies that you do like along with a couple of your favorite fruits, and gradually introduce new veggies weekly. Remember that it takes about 30 days for your taste buds to become used to a new food or a new way of eating a food, so don't give up.

Other components of **Fabulous Food** include grocery shopping around the store perimeter, avoiding packaged foods as much as possible, and reading labels when using packaged foods so you actually know what you are eating! If you don't know what the food ingredient is, don't eat it! Choosing healthy beverages is equally important, where water becomes your beverage of choice, along with unsweetened tea and coffee in moderation.

Eating a plant-based diet is the most important step in living a compassionate lifestyle. In addition, most people can benefit from the following supplements: probiotics, digestive enzymes, Vitamin B complex, Vitamin D, and omega-3 fatty acids in the form of flaxseed and raw nuts/seeds. Be sure to discuss the possible addition of these supplements with your healthcare provider.

Engaging in **Fantastic Fitness** has a myriad of health benefits, including weight control, as well as improved cognitive function, vascular stability, blood sugar levels, moods, and self-esteem. Plus, it can be fun, if we just engage in the right movements! I tell my patients that "when we stop moving our bodies, they slowly begin to die." I truly believe that when we move our bodies, we are telling them that we have not yet completed our tasks on this earth, and we need our bodies to move freely in order for us to continue our work unimpeded. When our bodies are fit, we not only gain longevity in life, but we establish an abundant quality of life that makes life worth living. After all, our goal in life is not just to live a long life, but to live a quality life for as long as we live. And, a quality life includes measures of health that are brought into being by keeping our bodies fit and moving.

What kind of activity is the best to do? The simple answer is any activity that we actually will do on a regular basis! We should find activities that are fun and bring happiness to our heart. We can incorporate joyful activity consistently into our everyday schedules. My favorite activity is to take long walks in nature; your favorite activity may be playing a soccer game. As long as we happily move our bodies, we will reap the advantages of **Fantastic Fitness**.

In addition, when we are at work, we can stand and walk around our desk if possible at least once hourly. We can stand when on the phone and at meetings as is practical. At home, we can get up at every commercial when watching TV, and walk around our chair where we are sitting. We can remember that frequent standing is good for our health, and thus avoid the "sitting disease" where we sit for too long and for too often, which can contribute to obesity and chronic disease.

Promoting **Festive Fun** in our lives brings a multitude of positive results, particularly in the areas of mental, physical, and emotional health. I heard someone say that children laugh about 300 times daily, and adults laugh 3 times daily. We should all ask ourselves, "What happens between ages 5 and 55 that causes our laughter to shut down?" The easy answer is, "Life happens." And, yes, life brings its challenges, but what would result if we attempted to return to the unabashed, abundant joy of a young child as often as possible? I have three young grandsons whose chuckles, giggles, and cackles can lessen and sometimes remove any troubles that I am feeling when I am in their magical presence. I venture to say that our lives would be immeasurably happier and our hearts sustainably lighter if we brought the abundance of laughter into our lives daily.

If you ever have the opportunity to participate in a Laughter Yoga class, google "laughter yoga" and you will find much information about how to incorporate a unique kind of laughter combined with exercise and deep breathing into your life. Laughter combined with movement and deep breathing increases oxygen delivery to your tissues, releases your feel good hormones, and helps you to let go of stress. The health benefits that you can receive from a Laughter Yoga class will be well worth your investigation!

We will discuss other aspects of **Festive Fun** that will assist us in coping with stress, including choosing nurturing thoughts and establishing a meditative and devotional practice, in future chapters.

Often, we know what we need to do to lower our risks for developing chronic diseases such as heart disease, diabetes, and cancer, but we continue to make unhealthy choices out of habit, addiction (do you realize that even thinking about eating sugar and fat can light up the same areas of the brain that cocaine and heroin do?), cultural and social pressures, and lack of self-love. It is possible to change habits, stop addictions, rise above unhealthy cultural and social pressures, and learn to love ourselves more. And changes don't have to occur overnight, but can take place in small increments over time that I like to call "baby steps."

For example, I often tell my patients to consider the "Zero Rule," which encourages them to celebrate for every 1 pound of body weight that they lose, they can take the "1" and place a "0" to the right of it, which gives them the number "10." I explain that when they lose "1" pound, they actually have taken the equivalent of "10" pounds of pressure off the joints of their lower back, hips, knees, ankles, and feet. Similarly, if they lose "10" pounds of body weight, they have taken the equivalent of "100" pounds of pressure off their lower body joints.

With the concept of baby steps in mind, I ask you to consider this week committing to one conscious choice (one baby step) from the list below, adding a new step weekly, and you will find that these baby steps, one-at-a-time, will warm your heart and recharge your health.

MEDICAL INSIGHT #3: EMBRACING COMPASSIONATE LIVING

Baby Steps for **Fabulous Food:**

1. Pack at least one lunch per week from home that includes some of your favorite healthy foods.

2. Eat an apple a day (keep fruit in your desk at work for a healthy snack).

3. Drink sparkling flavored water or water with lemon instead of diet soda or soda.

4. Substitute one healthy ingredient for a less healthy ingredient when cooking: i.e., Smart Balance non-dairy butter and non-dairy milk instead of dairy butter or margarine and milk, oatmeal instead of sugared cereal, agave instead of sugar, whole wheat flour or gluten-free flour instead of white flour, sourdough or rye bread instead of white bread.

5. Experiment with one day per week of meatless eating.

6. Share a meal when you eat out, or eat half of your meal and take the other half home.

7. Request low or no salt for your meal when you eat out.

8. Enjoy sorbet or fruit salad instead of a heavy dessert.

9. Drink water, then eat; or eat, then drink.

10. Eat mindfully using a smaller spoon and plate; chew each bite thoroughly before swallowing.

Three excellent resources to assist you along your journey of **Fabulous Food** are Kris Carr's www.kriscarr.com, and Colleen Patrick-Goudreau's www.the30dayveganchallenge.com, and the book by Neal D. Barnard, *21-Day Weight Loss Kickstart*.[4]

Baby Steps for **Fantastic Fitness:**

1. Find an activity that you like and then do it often (gardening, sports, walking, etc.).

2. Have a **Fantastic Fitness** buddy that you exercise with or who encourages you to exercise regularly.

3. Take the stairs instead of the elevator.

4. Park in the most distant parking spot at work.

5. Stand, instead of sit, for one-half of each work meeting; better yet, be the instigator for a walking work meeting as appropriate.

6. Do 5 minutes daily of desk aerobics (check out www.abeforfitness.com).

7. Walk around your TV chair instead of sitting in it during shows and/or commercials.

8. Walk daily with a family member or friend before work or after supper.

9. Stand at your work computer/desk periodically.

10. Use the employee or local gym for workouts/yoga classes/sporting activities.

Baby Steps for **Festive Fun**: (more explanation on these steps in future chapters)

1. Take 1 deep breath as often as you can.

2. Commit to 5-10 minutes of a morning or evening devotional/meditation practice.

3. Join a yoga, pilates, or tai chi class.

4. Take a TV holiday at least one day per week and substitute an activity that stimulates your body or brain.

5. Try a weekly meditation while walking.

6. Eat one meal weekly with mindfulness, chewing each bite at least 5 times.

7. Engage in belly laughter daily.

8. Treat yourself to a massage or reflexology appointment monthly.

9. Start a dream journal where you record and reflect upon your remembered dreams.

10. Increase restful sleep by using good sleep hygiene.

I like the quote from author and speaker Colleen Patrick-Goudreau, a leader in the compassionate lifestyle movement, that points out, "If we don't have time to be sick, then we have to make time to be well."[5] **Fabulous Food, Fantastic Fitness,** *and* **Festive Fun** *are abundant vehicles that can lead us down the exciting road of living a more compassionate life that will support us in gradually replacing love with fear, and in the process we will discover a healing of our heart and a transformation of our health.*

CHAPTER 4:

Love: Outshining the Shadows of Depression and Anxiety

After my hysterectomy at age 29, I felt like a cloud of depression descended on me. I honestly can say that I had never experienced what I would call clinical depression until that time. I suffered recurrent symptoms of sadness, irritability, sleep disruption, lack of motivation, inability to cry, and low to nonexistent levels of joy. I believe that the hormonal imbalances that resulted from my hysterectomy—discussed in Chapter 2—propelled me not only into physical symptoms but into emotional and mental imbalances as well. Fortunately, I had the strong support of my family, and caring for my young children and teaching music kept me busy and somewhat fulfilled, but I harbored an underlying daily depression that robbed me of a quality of life that I had previously known.

As my hormonal balances were corrected, my depression gradually resolved, but in its place I developed a terrifying new symptom: anxiety. This anxiety was more than normal concern about everyday circumstances that we all experience from time to time. This frightful anxiety that I experienced swept me up in its all-encompassing panic, and it began to accompany ordinary activities that I always had been able to do, but now wanted to avoid because they produced severe anxiety.

For example, I noticed suddenly that I did not like to be at heights or in small spaces. I wanted to avoid travel on boats or airplanes, and if I did find it absolutely necessary to travel, I wanted to make sure that I was close to a hospital, "just in case." I started feeling anxious about being alone with my young children because I feared that if I became ill while they were under my watch, I might not be able to care for them properly. I developed severe panic during recitals or concerts where I was performing or conducting, so much so that I felt faint, experienced heart palpitations, and barely restrained myself from bolting out of the room. I later learned that these symptoms were called "free floating anxiety," which was a perfect description of the myriad of anxiety and panic that I daily experienced.

As new anxieties continued to develop and I began to feel truly incapacitated to conduct my daily activities without severe anxiety accompanied by frequent panic attacks, I realized that I needed to get outside help. As I was contemplating what would be the best help for me to receive, I happened to walk into a bookstore, and my eye caught the title of a book on display, *Peace from Nervous Suffering* by Dr. Claire Weekes. As I quickly glanced through it, I immediately knew that Dr. Weekes was offering the help that I was seeking—

cognitive behavioral therapy for anxiety and panic attacks. I bought it and eagerly began to read and implement her advice, and my life began to change for the better. My panic attacks and severe anxiety gradually improved over a couple of months after implementing Dr. Weekes's recovery plan, which was nothing short of miraculous.

Once a person has experienced severe anxiety and panic attacks, he or she is more vulnerable to setbacks and returning panic attacks. Dr. Weekes's book also provides a plan to address setbacks and any returning panic attacks or lingering anxiety. The advice in her book is also excellent for persons who experience lower levels of chronic anxiety. Now, when I experience more common anxieties, I know what to do to quell the anxious thoughts before they reach a level of panic, thanks to the tools of cognitive behavioral therapy that I learned from Dr. Weekes's book. Over the years, I have shared many of these tools with my patients and referred them to cognitive behavioral therapy because I have found such benefit from this type of therapy for anxiety.

I do not believe that it was a coincidence that I developed depression, severe anxiety, and panic attacks at a time when my hormone levels had plummeted after my hysterectomy at age 29. I also know that I had very little love for myself at that time, because any love that I had for myself was constantly being overpowered by fear: fear that no matter how hard I tried, I couldn't seem to manage my anxiety; fear that I would never "get my life back again;" fear that I was "losing my mind;" fear that I was letting down my loved ones, and that they would leave me because of my illness; fear that I was not being a good enough mother; and on and on. In short, my life was ruled by fear, not empowered by love.

It is because of both my personal and professional experiences with depression and severe anxiety that I can say with certainty that these illnesses foster frightening, demoralizing, and paralyzing experiences that can rob us of the joy of living life. That is the shadow side.

However, because of my experiences, I have been able to shine a light into the shadows of depression and anxiety for many of my family members and my patients who have experienced these often debilitating illnesses. And, you will be able to do the same for others as you discover healing for yourself. We will be discussing in this chapter a number of ways to shine a light into the shadows of depression and anxiety that can help to illuminate our paths to wholeness and recovery.

The fourth chakra is the center of the heart, and the heart is symbolic of our center of emotions, particularly the emotion of love. In many ways, fear is just an absence of love. When we are able to replace fear with love, we find that we can begin to heal our hearts and transform our health.

In order to move from paralyzing fear to blissful love, whether caused by depression and/or anxiety, it is important to understand the causes of depression and anxiety. Although depression and anxiety are complex diseases that signify an imbalance in hormones and neurotransmitters, both depression and anxiety are accompanied by high levels of fear and low levels of self-love. Thus, when roots of fear and self-disdain are explored, we often notice an improvement in depression and anxiety. I have found both personally and professionally that a comprehensive approach to treating depression and anxiety—including medication as needed and appropriate cognitive and psychological therapies—may lead to greater and more lasting improvements for patients who suffer from depression and anxiety.

If you are suffering from depression or severe anxiety that is disrupting your life with fear and hopelessness, it is important for you to seek help from a healthcare professional as soon as possible. There are many pharmaceutical drugs that can be helpful. Treatment with pharmaceutical drugs is outside the scope of this book, so please discuss with a healthcare professional whether medication would be appropriate for you. Consider that medication may only be needed as a short-term therapy until you can implement long-term nutritional and cognitive behavioral therapies.

In addition to pharmaceutical treatment, several herbs have been shown to improve symptoms of both anxiety and depression. An herb that has been shown by scientific studies to benefit both depression and anxiety is Rhodiola.[1,2] You will want to discuss this option with your practitioner. As with any herbal supplement, you will want to obtain Rhodiola from a reputable source and take it as prescribed. Rhodiola is known to have little to no side effects, and can be taken for as long as is needed. Other herbs, such as SAMe and St. John's

Wort, have been shown to be helpful for depression, and herbs such as Passion Flower and Holy Basil have been shown to reduce anxiety.[3,4,5] Each person has a different response to medication, so be certain to discuss the potential use of these herbs with a healthcare professional.

A second option that you might want to consider as a solo treatment or as an adjunct to medication or herbal supplements for anxiety and/or depression is cognitive behavioral therapy. I highly recommend that if you or a loved one or friend suffers from the shadows of anxiety, panic attacks, and/or depression to seek cognitive behavioral counseling through a licensed counselor or psychologist. If face-to-face counseling seems too intimidating, you might want to consider online therapy at a website such as http:// counsellingresource.com/lib/therapy/service/live-online-therapy.

In addition to professional counseling, many excellent cognitive behavioral books can be helpful for persons who feel able to implement a recovery plan outlined in a book by a healthcare professional, without actually meeting with a healthcare professional in person or online.

Although the book that I mentioned above by Dr. Claire Weekes, *Peace From Nervous Suffering*, is now out of print, Dr. Weekes wrote a similar book, *Hope and Help for Your Nerves* that can be obtained online or at local bookstores.[6] You also can peruse through the self-help area of a local bookstore, library, or online bookstores and find other good cognitive behavioral therapy sources. The bottom line is to get the help and support that you need without delay. If you are currently paralyzed by fear and cannot move forward toward recovery, please engage the help of a friend of family member to assist you.

Additional therapies that have been shown to benefit both symptoms of depression and anxiety include engaging in **Fabulous Food**, **Fantastic Fitness**, and **Festive Fun** as discussed in Chapters 3 and 7, considering taking supplements such as Vitamin D, Vitamin B complex, and omega-3 fatty acids, exposing yourself to natural light or a light box, balancing your hormones, and abstaining from alcohol.

Two other excellent resources that I highly recommend to assist you in discovering healing from depression and anxiety include Dr. Andrew

Weil's comprehensive book, *Spontaneous Happiness*,[7] and Dr. Daniel Amen's revolutionary book, *Healing Anxiety and Depression*.[8]

Engage in the following daily cognitive behavioral therapies that will jumpstart you on your road to recovery.

MEDICAL INSIGHT #4: OUTSHINING THE SHADOWS OF DEPRESSION AND ANXIETY

1. Remember: anxious and depressed thoughts are just thoughts, not real truths or actions.

   There is no need to attach undue meaning to these thoughts. The more meaning that you attach to these thoughts, the more that these thoughts will continue to frighten you, and the more that you will continue to think them. Instead, each time that you have an anxious or depressed thought, first smile, and then remind yourself that it is only a thought. Visualize the thought floating through your heart rather than staying fixed within your heart.

2. When you have an anxious or depressed thought, ask yourself 2 questions:

1) Am I certain that this thought is 100%, completely true?

2) Does this thought bring out my highest self?

Likely your answer to both of these questions will be "No." Asking and answering these questions will help you to see that often anxious or depressed thoughts are untrue, bogus ideas that are highly unlikely to occur. Your answer of "No" will assist you in not attaching undue meaning to your anxious or depressed thoughts.

3. Practice taking the anxious or depressed thought and letting it go.

Imagine that you are writing the thought on a small piece of paper, and then placing the paper inside a balloon. Blow up the balloon, tie it, and then imagine that you are letting the balloon go gently into the air. Visualize your thought on the paper inside the balloon gently floating away. Take a deep relaxing breath, and see yourself as happy and well, living at the level of your highest self. Do this every time that the thought returns, remembering that it is just a thought, not a real truth or action. We will discuss more about choosing nurturing thoughts in Chapter 6.

4. Continue the "mirror work" that we discussed in Chapter 1.

One way to activate our fourth chakra so that loving thoughts can more habitually outshine fearful thoughts in our responses to the circumstances of our lives is to spend some time loving ourselves. By daily looking into a mirror and repeating, "I deeply love and approve of myself," we allow love to be dominant over fear in our lives.

5. Each day upon awakening, remember a time when you felt love and acceptance from another person, and now re-extend that same love and acceptance to yourself.

   As we practice replacing non-accepting fear with loving acceptance of ourselves and then expanding this love to others, we will discover that our depression and anxiety will lessen.

Working with a practitioner to implement appropriate medical treatments, cognitive behavioral therapies, and other lifestyle interventions can set us on a lifelong path of health. We will find that these steps will shine a light of love into our fearful shadows of depression and anxiety, and thus our hearts will begin to heal and our health will be transformed.

CHAPTER 5:

Truth and Forgiveness: Making Peace with Chronic Pain and Illness

After approximately two decades of practicing a compassionate lifestyle, I was diagnosed in early 2014 with multiple sclerosis (MS). For a number of months before my diagnosis, I had noticed that both of my feet and legs were developing almost constant symptoms of increasing numbness and tingling, so much so that I was finding it more difficult to drive or sit for periods of more than 30 minutes without my legs and feet becoming uncomfortably numb. I assumed that these symptoms were coming from a compressed nerve in my lower back, although I had not noticed any new lower back pain. I initially sought help from an osteopathic physician, and although my symptoms improved in the day or two after our sessions, they would gradually return in between my treatments.

My lower extremity numbness escalated to the point that I began to have both bowel and bladder hesitancy, so I was admitted to the hospital for emergency intervention and testing. Imaging of my thoracic spine showed abnormalities, and I was initially given the diagnosis of acute transverse myelitis—an inflammation of the central nervous system—since my age and presentation made it more unlikely that I had MS. I received 3 days of intravenous medications, and was discharged from the hospital feeling a little better and with the prognosis that my symptoms should continue to improve and perhaps even resolve over time.

However, my symptoms worsened over the next two months. I began having difficulty walking because of weakness in my legs and feet and developed problems with my balance. For the next three months, I continued to develop new symptoms weekly on top of the old ones. I experienced severe pain and abnormal sensation in my jaw, face, head, torso, and right shoulder, arm, and hand. I began to have intermittent blurry vision and pain in my parotid gland that made it painful to eat. I suffered itching over my entire back and scalp, and every time I bent my head forward, I felt an electrical shock sensation that travelled throughout my arms, torso, and legs. I always had been cold-natured, but now even mild elevations of temperatures seemed intolerable and increased my symptoms. The pain and disabling nature of my symptoms—now diagnosed by my neurologist as MS—in addition to my incapacitating fatigue, finally led me to take a medical leave of absence from my job as a physician.

From looking at the results of my blood work done in the hospital, you would have thought that I was the "picture of perfect health," with the exception of my Vitamin D level, which was so low that it was not even measurable. I knew that my Vitamin D level had been low in the past, and because I was aware that a low Vitamin D level could place me at a greater risk for developing many chronic diseases—since every cell in the body needs Vitamin D to function optimally—I had attempted repeatedly over a period of several years to take Vitamin D supplements. However, Vitamin D supplements, even at low doses, would oddly bring my myasthenic symptoms of generalized weakness out of remission, so I had been unable to take Vitamin D supplements, and my skin was rarely exposed to sunlight given my work schedule. I always advised my patients to know and keep their Vitamin D levels within an optimal range, but I felt helpless to raise my own Vitamin D level, given my inability to supplement or sun. Although I can't say that my low Vitamin D level caused me to develop MS, I can say that my low level increased my risk.

Most persons can tolerate Vitamin D supplements, but, as a result of my experience, if you have low levels of Vitamin D and cannot tolerate Vitamin D supplements, I highly recommend increasing your sun exposure or using a tanning bed if your daily schedule or geographic location does not allow adequate sunning to keep your levels optimal. You may ask, "But doesn't sunning or tanning bed use increase your risk for skin cancer?" The answer to that question is complex. Yes, the UVA and UVB rays that we get from the sun can increase our risk for developing certain types of skin cancer if we overdo it. In fact, any time you notice a tan, it tells you that your skin has been somewhat compromised as a result of sun exposure. However, most Vitamin D experts agree that 10-15 minutes of at least 40% body exposure in the midday sun several times weekly during the warmer months will increase your Vitamin D levels without putting you at significantly increased risk for developing certain skin cancers.[1] And, although some studies show that people who consistently use a tanning bed from young ages are at higher risk for developing melanoma—a potentially deadly form of skin cancer—other studies have shown that tanning beds can be used safely once or twice weekly during winter months when sunning is not possible or at any time in geographic areas where sun is not plentiful in order to maintain Vitamin D levels.[2] There even are tanning beds that expose you only to UVB rays—the rays that boost Vitamin D levels—and thus do not expose you to the UVA rays that contribute to tanning and increase skin damage and wrinkles.

It is important for you to educate yourself on Vitamin D first by having your 25-hydroxy Vitamin D blood levels checked, and then by determining in consultation with your physician how best to raise your levels if they are low, in order to diminish your risks for developing a chronic disease such as MS, or certain autoimmune diseases or cancers that are increasingly associated with low Vitamin D levels.

One of the things that I have learned from acquiring MS at this time in my life is that we cannot completely insulate ourselves from disease —whether it be MS or other neurological diseases, cancer, heart disease, or diabetes—but we can lower our risks for developing many diseases by making compassionate lifestyle choices. Although we are never guaranteed perfect health on this Earth, as I mentioned in Chapter 3, some diseases are virtually preventable with lifestyle changes, and other diseases have risks associated with them that can be lowered or eliminated. For example, stopping smoking will lower your risk for developing a myriad of diseases, both chronic and acute.

Fortunately, I am now on the gradual road that leads to improvement and recovery. Because I already was eating a plant-based diet—a diet that is recommended to assist in recovery from MS—I am a step closer to optimal health than if I had been eating a diet high in saturated fats derived from animal products.

Another philosophy that is healthy to adopt when we consider chronic pain and illness is that we should choose healthy lifestyles, not because we feel forced to deny ourselves anything fun or good in life in order to stay healthy, but because we enjoy giving to ourselves the gift of life and compassionate living through making healthy choices. If I had been eating healthfully and engaging in meditation and yoga only because my goal was to not develop disease, then I and others might say, "Well, what's the use? Dr. Bilhartz developed MS and she embraced a compassionate lifestyle. We might as well live as we please, because we are all going to die at some point anyway!" However, I have never participated in that way of thinking and regularly choose my lifestyle of abundant compassionate living because I love my body, appreciate what it does for me, and want to treat myself and all earthly creatures with the greatest kindness and respect. And, in the process of loving myself and others by making healthy lifestyle choices, I have received and will continue to receive blessings of a healthy mind, body, and spirit. Even though these choices do not ensure that I will be immune from developing disease, they make it less likely for me to be unhealthy, and more likely to recover from illness when it does develop. I believe that you will find the same to be true if you choose to make compassionate living a part of your daily life.

I think one of the best ways to learn from chronic disease and to make peace when we live with it is first to be able to accept the illness in all of it facets and expressions, not resisting or fighting it, but accepting it by asking ourselves: "What can I learn from this disease? Is it possible for me to view it as a blessing in disguise? How will my experience with this disease allow me to heal and to be a healer on this planet?" Dr. Judith Orloff, in her book *The Ecstasy of Surrender*, offers a "surrender affirmation" that speaks healing and restoration in the midst of pain and illness:

> I pledge to honor and love my body in sickness and in health. I pledge to keep surrendering negative thoughts and behaviors that sabotage my healing. During a health challenge I will keep surrendering pain and embrace gentleness, patience, and faith in the power of love.[3]

I have found that there is a difference between making a disease diagnosis the center of my identity versus seeking to discover what I can learn from the diagnosis and symptoms that are currently present in my life. For example, in making peace with chronic pain and illness, I believe that it is important to consider the physical, mental, and emotional aspects of our lives that may have contributed to the development of a specific disease at a particular time. Although we should never judge or blame ourselves for illnesses that we develop, if we treat only the outer symptoms of our illness without examining the current inner physical, mental, and emotional milieux of our lives that existed when we developed the illness, then we may miss the complete healing experience that is being offered to us if we can remain open to the potential lessons that can be learned from its experience.

For example, I believe that my low Vitamin D level may explain from the physical realm why I became so vulnerable to acquiring MS at this time in my life. And, as I have explored the mental and emotional aspects of the disease, or what we call the mind-body connection (we will discuss the mind-body connection more in Chapters 6 and 7), I can see that my life had been so full over the previous decade that perhaps my body just begged for a rest, even if this meant succumbing to illness in order to get the needed self-care my body desired.

Our fifth chakra reminds us that the energy from our throat center revolves around speaking our truth and yet refraining from judgment of ourselves or others if they do not hear or accept the truth as we see it. This means that making peace with chronic pain and illness often calls us to see our illness for what it is, and yet not judge ourselves or allow others' judgments of us to upset us. And, as we forgive ourselves for thinking that living with chronic illness means that we are less than we should be, and as we forgive others for comments or judgments toward us regarding our illness that we see as hurtful or critical, we set ourselves free from victimization and fear and move toward a greater love of ourselves and others, even in the midst of disease. This process allows our hearts to begin to heal and our health to journey toward transformation, even if we continue indefinitely to experience symptoms from our chronic illness.

One day, in the midst of some significant pain related to my MS, the thought came to me that "pain is my teacher, and love is my lesson." At first, I wasn't sure what this meant, but as I reflected on it, I realized that as we experience difficult chronic circumstances that challenge us to find ways to rise above them when possible or live within them when they cannot be changed, we become more compassionate and thus more able to help others in the process. Can you imagine if you had never experienced a challenge in life? You would have no knowledge or compassion to help others with their challenges! I will be a better doctor because I have experienced the topsy-turvy, uncertain, possibly incurable but manageable disease of MS, as much as I would have preferred not to have suffered the physical pain and disability that has accompanied my course of MS. As I allow myself to let my pain bring me into more love and compassion for myself and others, I can view my pain as a blessing in disguise, both for myself and for others. Although this is a difficult concept to embrace in the midst of pain, when we step back, we intuitively know this truth: as we find peace and love in the midst of chronic pain, our suffering takes on a higher purpose, and thus is never in vain.

Our hearts become more fully whole and our health more deeply transformed as we realize that part of the reason that we exist on this earth is to serve as healers for ourselves and others. We discover the healer that is innately present in us as we allow ourselves to move from fear to love, even in the midst of our current health challenges.

Consider the following approaches to bring yourself into greater truth and forgiveness, as you discover ways to make peace with your chronic pain and illness.

MEDICAL INSIGHT #5: EMBRACING TRUTH AND FORGIVENESS AS WE MAKE PEACE WITH CHRONIC PAIN AND ILLNESS

1. Many chronic diseases can be improved and sometimes even resolved through healthy lifestyle choices. Contemplate how you might better educate yourself on your particular disease and its possible beneficial treatments by researching and reading credible sources. Work with your physician to maximize your health through an integrative approach to managing your chronic illness. This includes doing everything that is within your control to transform your health, including choosing healthy food and daily movement, stopping smoking, limiting or eliminating alcohol and stimulants, embracing truth and forgiveness, and reducing stress through meditation and nurturing thoughts (more about this in Chapters 6 and 7).

When you take charge of your life in the areas that you can control, you will find that you will feel more empowered and optimistic, your coping and energy levels will increase, and your pain—mental, physical, and emotional—will decrease. And with these changes, you possibly will be able to reduce or even eliminate your need for prescription medications, which although helpful and even necessary at times, can have risks that may outweigh their benefits if taken in higher doses over longer periods of time.

2. Ask your physician to check your levels of Vitamin D, Vitamin B12, and folate; hormones (including sex and thyroid hormones); and standard blood panels. Often, tweaking these levels as indicated can improve or eliminate many of your symptoms. Some physicians are not versed in testing and adjusting hormone levels, so if your labs appear normal and your doctor does not see any other medical reason why you are having your current symptoms, consider getting a second opinion from an integrative physician as discussed in Chapter 2.

Get adequate sleep. For most people, this means 7-8 hours nightly, and often more if you have a chronic illness. Practicing good sleep hygiene will enable you to sleep deeply and awaken rested. Proper sleep hygiene includes a good mattress, proper room temperature, a darkened room, no caffeine after lunch, smaller meals at dinner, no alcohol in the evening (although alcohol may make you temporarily drowsy, it interrupts deep sleep), daily exercise, no computer/TV within 1-2 hours of bedtime, and bedtime rituals such as meditating or a warm bath. For short periods of time, there are several supplements that can assist you in obtaining better sleep that can be taken in consultation with your physician, including Valerian,[4] Melatonin, and Progesterone.

Taking charge of our health by learning about our disease and its treatment options, by making compassionate choices, and by living in truth and forgiveness will help us to find peace, even in the midst of our chronic illness. We find that when we can lovingly accept our symptoms while simultaneously embracing complete health, love will gradually replace fear, and we will heal our hearts and transform our lives.

CHAPTER 6:

Clarity: Choosing Nurturing Thoughts

I n 1999, scientist Dr. Candace Pert released her landmark book, *Molecules of Emotion: The Science Behind Mind-Body Medicine,* and began a whole new discussion on a field called psychoneuroimmunology.[1] The persuasive message of her book—that the mind-body connection played an important but often missing link in the treatment of illness and disease—became a propelling force in my life as I began to consider changing my career from music to medicine. Deep down inside of me I recognized a passionate desire that originated from a power much greater than myself to bring this growing conundrum of likely healing knowledge to others.

"Psychoneuroimmunology" is a long word, but it simply means that thoughts released in our minds trigger emotional reactions that in turn cause our body to release chemicals and hormones that control our pleasure centers and can produce positive or negative health effects. Dr. Pert's research, based on biomolecular cell behavior, demonstrated objectively that there indeed was an integrated communication network between our minds and bodies. She detailed this psychoneuroimmunological response in the body by scientifically demonstrating that specific thoughts propel the body to create certain amino acids called neuropeptides that then carry chemical messages from the brain to receptors in cells all over the body. These neuropeptides serve as the key that then unlocks the cell to release more chemicals that control cell behavior and ultimately the health of our body. Amazingly, our nervous, endocrine and immune systems appear to be joined in an intricate network of body responses that actually begin with our thoughts.

Think about it like this. Neuropeptides released as a result of a particular thought can signal the volume and speed of our blood flow by causing the cells to release certain chemicals that then contribute to blood vessel constriction or dilation. Thus, when we are afraid or under stress, we can turn "white as a ghost" when a fearful thought triggers certain blood vessels to constrict, or "red as a beet" when the vessels in our face dilate in response to a denigrating thought triggered by an embarrassing moment. Neuropeptide release prompted by stressful or anxious thoughts can affect virtually every cell and organ in our body, causing our hearts to race, our guts to feel tight, our breaths to become more shallow, our legs to shake, our heads to feel "light," and our hands to become clammy.

So if our thoughts can elicit responses in our bodies, what kinds of specific adverse effects can stressful thoughts have on our health? For starters, when we feel stressed, we release higher levels of a chemical called cortisol (briefly discussed in Chapter 2), and while cortisol is an important hormone whose function is to assist our body in functioning more optimally when we are under duress, this "fight or flight" response was only meant to be used intermittently for short periods of time as needed. Cortisol's optimal release should occur during short periods of stress and early in the morning, with gradual lowering of levels as the day goes on so that sleep can occur at night. Chronically elevated cortisol levels contribute to insomnia, lower immune function, and less focus, along with increased blood sugar, blood pressure, inflammation, stomach acid, cholesterol, heart rate, and irritability.

In contrast, how do more relaxed thoughts trigger health enhancing responses in our bodies? With more peaceful thoughts, instead of activating our "fight and flight" system, we set into motion our "rest and digest" system. Our cortisol levels drop, so our blood sugar levels drop. When cortisol levels drop as the day goes on, our melatonin levels begin to increase in the evening. Melatonin is what causes us to fall asleep and to engage in less interrupted, deeper sleep. Our digestive system works more optimally so we have fewer symptoms of bloating, gas, and constipation. Our heart rate slows and we breathe more deeply, which optimally oxygenates our tissues and blood. We release more oxytocin—our "feel good" hormone—and dopamine and serotonin levels increase, so we feel happier, less moody, and more relaxed. We have greater interest in sex, and our bodies cooperate to make sex more pleasurable for us. All of these healthy responses occur when our body is operating in its "rest and digest" mode.

Although the idea that our attitudes, beliefs, and thought patterns can affect our health for better or worse was not new, the scientific evidence that sprung from Dr. Pert's groundbreaking research in psychoneuroimmunology stimulated further study and interest on the part of scientists and physicians in the area of mind-body medicine. I became so mesmerized by the topic of mind-body medicine that I voraciously devoured everything that I could read about the subject. Some of my favorite books that addressed the importance of choosing mindful thoughts that in turn could nurture our body's health included Daniel Amen's *Change Your Brain, Change Your Life*,[2] Herbert Benson's *The Relaxation Response*,[3] Deepak Chopra's *Perfect Health: The Complete Mind/Body Guide*,[4] Wayne Dyer's *Change Your Thoughts—Change Your Life*,[5] Jon Kabat-Zinn's *Full Catastrophe Living: Using the Wisdom of Your*

Body and Mind to Face Stress, Pain, and Illness,[6] Christiane Northrup's *Women's Bodies, Women's Wisdom,*[7] and Mona Lisa Schulz's *Awakening Intuition: Using Your Mind-Body Network for Insight and Healing.*[8]

One of the basics that we need to understand in the field of mind-body medicine is that all of us face challenging circumstances, but how much these circumstances affect our health is based on what we think about the event and whether or not we perceive it as stressful. One of the best books that I have read on the subject of how our bodies perceive stress is Richard Carlson's book, *Don't Sweat the Small Stuff… and It's All Small Stuff,* which reminds us that most of life's events that we perceive as stressful actually are not worth us sweating over. Often these events never even befall us, and even if they do, they usually are not nearly as devastating as we might have originally anticipated.[9] Carlson's book reminds us that the thoughts that we think about life's happenings matter, and that if we can reframe adverse circumstances from being perceived stressors instead to disguised blessings, we will remain happier people and our health will flourish rather than flail. In other words, building optimal health using our own nurturing thoughts is actually under our control.

We likely can agree that nurturing thoughts can benefit our health, but it can be more difficult to learn how to choose those thoughts that will move our body toward healing and more optimal function. One of the first books that I read that assisted me in learning to release non-productive and non-nurturing thoughts was Louise Hay's book *You Can Heal Your Life* that I mentioned in Chapter 1.[10] You might enjoy reading excerpts from this book daily as you begin to clean out unwanted and unneeded thoughts from your mind and replace them with loving, productive thoughts that nurture your health.

We might argue that it can be difficult if not seemingly impossible to control our thoughts, but the truth is that we can learn to be the masters of our thoughts with practice. I like the metaphor of a conveyor belt on which our thoughts travel. We have the choice to select off of the conveyor belt any thought that would be beneficial to our health, and to leave on the conveyor belt any thought that does not serve our highest health. We can develop a keen mental perception and understanding of our thoughts, realizing that thoughts are just thoughts and truly can be changed as we become aware of them and desire to make changes.

Our body's energy center that aids us in finding clarity of thought is located just above the area between the brows at the place of the "third eye." This is the sixth chakra that allows us to see truth and to know purity of thought. Some of the best ways to shape our thoughts toward healing are through loving ourselves unconditionally, living fearlessly, practicing forgiveness, and releasing non-nurturing thoughts as we accept nurturing ones. Chapter 7 will address additional ways to practice the release of non-nurturing thoughts. And over time, we will move our thoughts from health-depleting to health-repleting ones.

Try the following practices that will provide further clarity in helping you to release your stressful thoughts and reshape them into joyous, health-enhancing ones.

MEDICAL INSIGHT #6:
CHOOSING NURTURING THOUGHTS

1. Apply the Baby Steps approach that we discussed in Chapter 3 to assist you in recognizing non-nurturing thoughts quickly and discovering fun ways to reframe them.

    First, set an intention that you want to recognize and reframe non-health enhancing thoughts.

    Second, set aside a few minutes daily to begin a journal where you determine to write down 10 of your most repeated daily thoughts.

    Third, reflect on each thought, asking yourself if the thought is worthy of your thought time in that it is health-increasing, or is it a worry thought that is not worth your time because it is health-decreasing.

    Finally, reframe each non-nurturing thought as you ask yourself the following questions: Is this thought a true thought? How can I change it into a nurturing thought that reflects clarity of thought and truth?

    Now rewrite the reframed thought by using the following two questions to assist you in changing a worry thought into a health enhancing one:

    1) How can you see the glass as half full rather than half empty?;

    2) How can you take a lemon and use it to make lemonade?

Reflect on this new health enhancing thought repetitively throughout your day until it g r a d u a l l y replaces your old non-nurturing thought.

For example, let's say that one of your written thoughts is, "I am overweight and unattractive." Ask yourself if this is a true thought. You may immediately want to respond with a "yes," but I want you to think more deeply. Find something about yourself that is attractive, such as your eyes, hair, skin, hands, or inner beauty. Let's say that y o u remember that your inner beauty shone recently when you demonstrated kindness to a coworker or family member. Now, revisit your thought and realize that "I am unattractive" is not a completely true statement. Next, reframe the thought, "I am overweight" to create a health enhancing thought such as, "I weigh more than I want today, but I am actively working to achieve my ideal weight by making compassionate choices daily. I choose to celebrate the things that are attractive about me and love myself unconditionally during this process." Lovingly speak this thought to yourself repetitively throughout your day as you establish a new, healthful way of thinking.

2. Make a game of identifying your ANT thoughts as discussed by Dr. Daniel Amen in his book that I mentioned earlier in this chapter, *Change Your Brain, Change Your Life*. ANTs are Automatic Negative Thoughts that deplete our health.[11] ANTs include:

- Fortune-telling: I will never be happy.

- Labeling: I am always a failure.

- Blame: If my parents hadn't gotten a divorce, I wouldn't always be so unhappy.

- Guilt beating: I am constantly a disaster.

- Mind reading: I don't know why they never like me.

Note that the one consistent word in the above ANT statements is an absolute such as "never, always, or constantly." Any time that you use these absolute words, you can rest assure that the statement is not completely true, and thus can be reframed.

Practice recognizing and then laughing any time that you think an ANT thought. Laughing at the thought helps it dissipate, and allows you to be open to reframe it into a health enhancing one.

As we become more aware of our thoughts, we will likely notice that most of them throughout the day are based on fear: fear that we are not enough, fear that others will hurt us, and fear that negative circumstances will come our way. We can begin to reframe the fearful thoughts into ones where we love ourselves unconditionally enough to forgive ourselves, love others compassionately enough to stop judging them, and love the Divine enough to trust that good always comes our way, even if it seems "bad" at the time (more about this in Chapter 8). As we joyfully reframe our stressful, unhealthy thoughts into ones that are productive and conducive to healthy living, fear will give way to love, and we will begin to heal our hearts and transform our health, one thought at a time.

CHAPTER 7:

Guidance: Finding Your Center

I shared in Chapter 1 how I learned very early on that I felt the need to prove to myself and others that I was worthy of acceptance and love. What went along with my pursuit of achievement and perfection was worry accompanied by its underlying base of fear. I daily experienced all-encompassing fears, such as fear that I was not enough and fear that I might disappoint myself and others, as well as day-to-day fears that I wouldn't ace the next test or people wouldn't like me.

I also told my story in Chapter 4 about how later in my life I developed something more severe than everyday intermittent worries—free floating anxiety and panic attacks—and learned from that experience that as I allowed fearful thoughts to seep deeply into all crannies of my life, the fear began to so overtake me that my mind became almost continually flooded with a myriad of anxious thoughts. Once I used the tools of cognitive behavioral therapy to assist me in letting my thoughts float through me rather than being caught up in their drama, I began to recover from my severe anxiety. Becoming a practicing student of cognitive therapy benefitted me in not only helping my severe anxiety to dissipate, but in the process I discovered that I could use some of the same cognitive behavioral techniques to address my day-to-day worries.

Don't misunderstand me. I do not believe that worry always leads to panic attacks, or that severe anxiety has only one cause, and that cause is chronic worry. We likely can trace the roots of most illnesses to combinations of mind, body, and spirit imbalances. I mentioned in Chapter 4 that part of what I believe propelled me into severe anxiety and panic attacks was the hormonal imbalance that I experienced after my hysterectomy at age 29. However, physical causes of disease do not preclude mind and spirit contributors, including, for me, chronic worry that made it easier for my mind to be thrust into the arms of severe anxiety. And, as I continued to utilize the tools of cognitive behavioral therapy to bring resolution to my severe anxiety, I also gleaned assistance in tackling my habits of chronic worry.

For about a decade between my mid-thirties to mid-forties, I used cognitive behavioral therapy to assist my thoughts of daily worry to flow through me rather than getting stuck in the quagmire of my mind and body where the worry thoughts could wreak havoc on a peaceful daily existence of trust in the Divine. However, in my mid-forties, I discovered that there was an additional helpful tool that I had been unaware of that, with its use, could radically change my approach to dealing with chronic worry.

In short, I joined a yoga class in my town that met three times weekly. I joined the class in order to reduce my intermittent low back pain, but found that the deep breathing that we did throughout the class was a great stress buster. I would leave the class so refreshed that I noticed I would continue to breathe deeply for about an hour after I left. I also discovered that when I began to feel stressed during the day, if I would breathe more deeply, I would feel an almost immediate relaxation response and an amazingly efficient release of stressful thoughts and circumstances.

I began to practice my yoga postures daily at home, sometimes adding deep breathing and relaxation tapes while doing the postures, and thus my "meditation" practice began. I found it very exciting to learn that I actually had the power to lower my stress levels with regular daily meditation. In fact, the more that I engaged in daily meditation, not only were my stress and anxiety levels notably more manageable, I found myself embarking on a new journey that gradually began to move me further away from chronic fear and worry into love and acceptance.

My husband's interest in meditation became piqued about the same time as mine did, and so we began to explore various forms of meditation together. Early on, we used guided meditations that included affirmations and beautiful imagery to engage us in quieting our minds. One of our favorite series of relaxation and meditation CDs included guided imagery meditations called "Healthjourneys" that were produced by Belleruth Naparstek.[1] Over subsequent years, we continued to use guided imagery, but began to add a nightly meditation to our morning practice, and to experiment with other types of meditation practices including The Chopra Center's meditations with Deepak Chopra, David Simon, Oprah Winfrey, and Davidji;[2] "Mindfulness Meditation" with Jon Kabat-Zinn;[3] and Osho's "Active Meditations.[4]

Many meditative practices will offer the novice student some initial instruction, followed by a guided or unguided meditation. Most meditations are designed where the participant will be sitting or in a comfortable position, but some meditations are prescribed to be done while walking. Music often will accompany the meditation. Unguided meditations may or may not have accompanying music, and likely will be preceded by brief instruction and then silence so that the participant can meditate without further outside intervention or instruction. Guided meditations usually have musical accompaniment, and the instructor will offer thoughts, images, prayers, and affirmations to be considered by the participant during the time of meditation. With both types of meditation, the participant is encouraged to be quiet and receptive, and to allow thoughts outside of the topic of the meditation to float through the mind without becoming fixed on them.

The ultimate goal of meditation is to quiet the mind into silence, peace, and receptivity, although if this does not happen, the participant is encouraged not to dwell on the goal of meditation, but just to enjoy the now moment however it presents itself. A multitude of medical studies have demonstrated that practices of meditation and devotion can lower one's blood pressure, diminish anxiety, promote well-being, and even quell chronic pain and disease.[5,6] Professor George Jelinek, author of *Overcoming Multiple Sclerosis,* states, "There are now over 1500 papers in the medical literature on the health benefits of meditation."[7]

Initially, I loved my daily time of meditation because it allowed me to calm my mind and release stressful thoughts. Most persons experienced in meditation explain that as you become still and quiet your mind, you enter into the "sweet spot" deep within the center of your being where you become open to receiving your inner guidance. The concept of "inner guidance" was intriguing to me, because I came from a long line of women who set aside time daily for "devotions"—time where you prayed and read Sacred Scripture and sought outside help and peace from the Divine. I had taken the time daily for devotions since I was in my teens, and this practice had been and continues to be very beneficial to my spiritual growth and life's interactions. However, the idea that I might have an intuitive inner guidance resonated strongly with me, as I began to see the Divine Spirit as an innate part of my inner being that moved within me to shape my thoughts and actions, rather than just an outside power reigning over me.

As my meditation and devotional practices deepened and I more consciously connected with the Sacred Divine, I found that I began to learn more about myself and what thoughts and actions I needed to embrace in order to live at the level of my "higher self"—that self which makes wise and loving choices—and what triggers I needed to reframe in order to live more optimally in love and wisdom. Over time, the moments that I spent in meditation—breathing deeply, relaxing my mind, resonating peace and love, and allowing myself to "be" rather than "do"— gradually moved beyond the several-minute daily practice and began to transform my thoughts and actions during my other waking hours. The power that I found in choosing my thoughts during meditation assisted me in choosing my thoughts throughout the day. I found that my new, nurturing thoughts helped to shift and shape my emotions and actions in all of my activities, and this Guidance led me to experience unparalleled Joy, Love, and Peace.

Remember our discussion in the previous chapters about living a compassionate lifestyle and the importance of choosing our thoughts carefully? I believe that mindfulness always matters, whether it is with choosing **Fabulous Food**, **Fantastic Fitness**, or **Festive Fun** including healthful thoughts. Our wise choices and thoughts will always nurture a return to our Center, where Guidance is continuously available if we ask and then allow it to come. Meditation and devotion are tools that can assist us to remember our higher nature, and then daily to live from that guiding center in our thoughts and actions.

The seventh energy center is described as our crown chakra, and is located at the top of our head. In many ways, our crown chakra represents the culmination of all of our energy centers in the body. The seventh chakra energy opens us to the inner guidance of our spiritual self, and always encourages us to awaken to the Divine. By reminding us of our spiritual nature, it counterbalances our first chakra that challenges us to accept ourselves in all of our humanness. When we find ourselves living more and more from our higher nature, we enter into a world of miracles, happiness, and unlimited serendipity!

This way of walking in Beauty and Love sounds wonderful, but you may wonder, "Is this possible for me?" My answer is a resounding, "Yes!" Let's explore the Guidance to living life at the level of our highest self that can be fostered through the following Baby Step approach to meditation and devotion.

MEDICAL INSIGHT #7:
FINDING CENTERED GUIDANCE THROUGH A PRACTICE OF MEDITATION AND DEVOTION

1. Set an intention to begin a daily practice of meditation and devotion for 30 days. After the 30 days are up, you can evaluate its benefits and determine whether you wish to continue the practice. The practice will be most effective if you can set aside in a quiet space a minimum of 10 minutes twice daily where you will engage in the practice. However, the important thing is to be creative and make it work for you, even if this means practicing for a shorter period of time or less frequently, and incorporating other family members into the practice as needed.

2. A suggested outline for a daily practice would include reading a page or two from a favorite author, a short devotional, or a portion of Sacred Scripture that is of your choosing. Follow this reading with a prayer and a short guided or mindfulness meditation.

3. If you are novice to meditation, for starters, I would recommend using a guided meditation; you may download many for free off of the internet or purchase a CD from some of the leaders in

meditation that I mentioned earlier in this chapter. Experiment with a variety of meditations, and use the ones that resonate with your spirit and personality. You may find that you will enjoy a variety of meditations, or you may want to settle in with a particular one that stimulates you to practice it daily.

4. Praise yourself for any amount of discipline that you establish, and avoid berating yourself if you miss a session or day. You will find that your body begins to crave the peace and quiet of the meditative experience as much as it does the results of higher self living, and will gently guide you to continue your practice when possible.

The ultimate purpose of meditation and devotion is to enable us to lovingly experience our higher self and the Sacred Divine, and then to translate those experiences into service of lovingkindness to the world. Our universal purpose on this earth is to receive healing for ourselves, and then to pass this healing on to others. Let's begin to seek ways that we can live this purpose—at our job, with friends and family, and in our community and beyond. We will find that meditation and devotion will open us up to a fearless world of Infinite Possibilities where love can heal our hearts and transform our lives daily. Let's enjoy our blessed life that is always available to us at our choosing!

CHAPTER 8:

The Flow:
Reframing the
Impostors of Good
Luck, Bad Luck

I have written most of this book while on medical leave as I journey through the recovery process that goes along with my recent diagnosis of MS. This diagnosis already has given me an even deeper focus on the way that I view the world and frame health. I cannot tell you how to live your life; all I can do is to share my experiences and knowledge with you, and hope that you will take this information and use it for good in your life. My desire is that your motivation for healthy living will not come from fear, but will spring from love for yourself. We cannot be assured that our health will always be optimal, even with healthy lifestyle choices. However, we can lower our risks for major diseases and common illnesses, and increase our ability to rebound from illness, by choosing compassionate living. And, making compassionate choices brings healing to our hearts and transformation to our health when we choose wise living out of love for ourselves and others, rather than out of duty or drudgery.

I believe that every part of our body is interconnected, including all parts of our physical, mental, and spiritual natures. When the energy chakras in our bodies are seen as individual units, they become stagnant rather quickly, just as a body of water becomes immobile with no inflow or outflow. Chakras produce their greatest energy when they are interconnected by an unimpeded energy flow that cycles through them. At any point, the energy can be blocked. The key is to keep our energy areas open so that the "chi," or life force, can continue to circulate freely. This leads to optimal mental, physical, and emotional health.

An old parable tells the story of an aged man who had one horse and one son. One day, the horse ran away and the neighbors chattered, "Your horse ran away. What bad luck!" The old man replied, "Good luck, bad luck, who can tell? It is what it is. All I know is that my horse is gone." The next night, the man's horse returned along with twelve new horses. Again, the neighbors gathered, but this time, they said, "You now have thirteen horses. What good luck!" But the old man replied, "Good luck, bad luck, who can tell? It is what it is. All I know is that I now have thirteen horses." The next week, while the man's son was breaking in one of the horses, he fell and broke both of his legs. The neighbors again commented, "What bad luck!" The old man responded, "Good luck, bad luck, who can tell? It is what it is. All I know is that my son has two broken legs." Two weeks later, the government forcibly removed all able-bodied men from the village, since the country had declared war. The old man's son was not removed because both of his legs were broken. The neighbors cackled, "What good luck. Your son did not have to go to war." And the old man replied, "Good luck, bad luck, who can tell? It is what it is. All I know is that my son did not go to war."[1]

The reason that I share this story with you in a book that provides suggestions toward optimal health is that it reminds us that most often, we see illness as something that is bad, and we want its pain and inconvenience to go away as soon as possible. I encourage you to consider another way of viewing illness: begin to discover moments, even if they are fleeting, when you can direct your thoughts to help you reframe and embrace illness as a disguised blessing. When we are willing to see the ideas of "good luck, bad luck" for the impostors that they are, and that perceived "luck" always comes from the vantage point of the observer, illness can lead us to a flow of greater self-awareness and love, for ourselves and others. The British poet Rudyard Kipling says it well in his poem, *If*: "If you can meet with Triumph and Disaster, and treat those two impostors just the same...."[2]

The longer that I live, the more that I am compelled to live my life in the ever-renewing stream of love and forgiveness, to show compassion for myself and others, and to find joyful ways of being and doing on this earth. Living life in acceptance and gratefulness for the present moment exactly as it presents itself opens the door for the circulation of lovingkindness, first to ourselves and then to others. *New York Times* best-selling author Marianne Williamson simply states this wisdom of the practice of lovingkindness:

> Knowing who you are and why you came here—that you are a child of God and that you came here to heal and be healed—is more important than knowing what you want to do. What you want to do is not the important question. The question to ask is, 'When I do anything, how should I do it?' And the answer is, 'Kindly.'[3]

I had a recent mystical experience that demonstrates beautifully the deep truth that the flow of love has the ability in every situation to trump fear, and with that love our hearts are healed and our health is transformed. In this transformative process, we then are freed to be of greater service to this world.

One morning while standing at my printer, retrieving a paper, I spontaneously began to feel a wave of warmth wash over me that began with my head and slowly moved throughout my body to my feet. After my recent diagnosis with MS, now when I feel a new neurological sensation, I often am quick to react with concern that I may be developing a new MS symptom, but this feeling was distinctly different from an isolated neurological symptom because it was accompanied by the awareness that this warmth was not a symptom of MS but was the presence of Love, and as it washed over me, all fear was replaced by love. At the same instant that I felt the sensation and awareness of the power of Love, I heard in my mind the words to a song written by singer and composer Rickie Byars Beckwith, "We let the Love wash over us...."[4] I also began to envision in my mind's eye many scenarios in my life where I had felt fear, and I realized that I no longer felt any fear surrounding those circumstances, but only a wash of Love. I even recall thinking, "I could hold a scorpion and not be afraid!" That's a pretty amazing thought for me, since I have lived most of my life in New Mexico and Texas, and scorpions abound in these areas! (Needless to say, they have never been my most cherished arthropod ever since I was stung by one at a summer camp when I was about 12 years old.)

The "Love-Wash" experience, as I now refer to it, left me with a profound sense of overriding peace and joy, and an abiding knowledge that it truly was possible to reframe or even initially view all of life's experiences as sacred ones, if love rather than fear was the overriding emotion. Envision, for example, how our health would change if we no longer felt the need to defend ourselves at others' expense, if we went with the flow of life with trust and gusto, if we let go of some of our greatest fears with finality and commitment, and if we laughed and loved ourselves and others more. How much healing would our hearts experience if we sang instead of fussed, if we smiled instead of frowned, if we laughed instead of hollered, and if we let go of our small world views and let the Divine lead us to grander visions of life and love?

My message in this book is that optimal health is possible, but "optimal health" in its most sacred definition doesn't necessarily equate with having no health issues. In contrast, in this body, on this earth, we will be presented with health challenges, likely intermittently and perhaps chronically throughout life, but in the facing of these challenges and taking full responsibility for them, we have the capacity to wisely choose lovingkindness and compassionate living, including **Fabulous Food**, **Fantastic Fitness**, and **Festive Fun**. We are empowered as we take full responsibility for our health issues, no longer blaming others or our circumstances for our current health status. We can educate ourselves about our illnesses and thus select healthcare providers with whom we feel comfortable, who honor our intuitive knowledge about our bodies, and who treat the body, mind, and spirit as an integral whole. We have the autonomy to select healing thoughts, and to center and recenter ourselves throughout the day and night as we seek guidance from a Higher Power. We can let go of nonproductive judgments about ourselves and others, seek and speak our truth with kindness, and embrace love and forgiveness for ourselves and others. In short, we can choose to live at the level of our highest calling with full awareness as often as is possible while living, moving, and breathing in a human body. And as we allow ourselves to go freely with the flow of life, fear is replaced by love, and we ultimately access the healing for our hearts and transformation of our health that was always within us, just waiting to be discovered.

One way for us to enter into life's unimpeded flow of bountiful blessings and optimal health is to become aware of any blockages or impedances that prevent us from experiencing our fullest flow of energy. The following activities are valuable tools to assist you in removing these blockages and tuning into your highest level of physical, mental, and spiritual energy. I recommend using them daily or as often as possible, in order to enhance your health and wholeness.

MEDICAL INSIGHT #8: ENTERING INTO THE FLOW OF LIFE

1. "Increasing Energy Flow" meditation:

   Set aside at least 10 minutes during your daily meditation/devotional time for this guided meditation. You might want to turn on a background noise such as an ocean sound or fan. Then, get into a comfortable position, and take several deep breaths. With each inhalation, envision that you are taking Love and Health into your body; with each exhalation, see yourself letting out any thoughts or feelings that are non-nurturing.

Begin to visualize your body, starting with the area of the first chakra at the base of your spine. Say out loud or to yourself, "I am safe and secure." Imagine the power of Love warming and filling the first chakra area, noting that this warmth gradually clears all impedances from that area. See any energy that was stagnant as now able to flow freely to the second chakra. Some people find that visualizing Love as a powerful Light is very helpful.

Repeat the same visualization for subsequent chakras, while spending a minute or two envisioning warming Love and Light filling each area. With each chakra, repeat and reflect on the following phrases:

- Second chakra: "Life is a Pleasure."

- Third chakra: "I Have All that I Need."

- Fourth chakra: "I Am Loving to Myself and Others."

- Fifth chakra: "I Speak the Truth and Listen Without Judgment."

- Sixth chakra: "I See Clarity In All Things."

- Seventh chakra: "I Am Guided By A Higher Power."

When you have finished the seventh chakra visualization, visualize the energy now that is flowing from the first to the second to each chakra without interruption all the way to the seventh chakra, and then returning to the first chakra to recirculate continuously throughout the chakras with a calm, easy, moving flow.

When you are ready to end the meditation, take several deep breaths as you did at the beginning of the meditation.

Finish your meditation by repeating several times the phrase: "Love Trumps Fear in My Life Today."

Throughout the day, whenever you have a moment or feel the need to recenter yourself, take several deep breaths, visualize warm healing Love and Light flowing throughout your body, and repeat: "Love Trumps Fear in My Life Today."

This powerful guided meditation can be repeated in all or in part in any place, at any time, or during any situation to reestablish your energy flow, and bring your heart and health into a receptivity of optimal wellness.

2. Enter into the flow of self-reflection as you spend a few minutes each day writing in your journal about situations in your life where you were able to treat the impostors of "good luck, bad luck" or "triumph and disaster" just the same. How did an event that appeared as "bad luck" at the time become a blessing in disguise? When you experienced a moment of triumph or disaster in your life, how were you able to take it in stride, remaining thankful in both cases, knowing that all things can work for good as you allow and reframe them?

One of my favorite movie lines comes from the movie "Stranger Than Fiction."[5] The lead character in the movie, Harold Crick, played by Will Ferrell, is an IRS auditor who lived his life out of habit, fear, and drudgery until one day he discovered that he was likely going to die very soon. This realization propelled Harold to "go for broke" and decide to live passionately what was left of his life, with love and abandon. His change of heart was reflected by the line, "Harold Crick lived his life"—a meaningful play on words that life is meant to be lived joyfully in the thrill of each moment, and when we succeed in doing this, we truly "live." This is the choice that comes to each of us in our life moment by moment, and we have the autonomy to embrace life in all of its exciting, full serendipity with joy and love, or hide from life out of fear of what might happen if we allow its full experience to circulate through us. As I have reflected on this movie line,

I have discovered that I want to be able to say in this moment and throughout the rest of my life on this earth that "Patty Bilhartz lived her life." I intuitively know that if I "live my life" in lovingkindness both for myself and others, fear will continue to pale in comparison to love, and my heart and health will experience healing and transformation beyond my wildest dreams. My deepest desire is that you will join me in this incredible journey of life as we continue to find wholeness in the power of love.

EPILOGUE:

Join Our Community

N ow that you've read the book, we invite you to join our community and share with others who are discovering the joy of living compassionately in a nurturing environment. This is a community where we relish autonomy as we take loving responsibility for our compassionate life's choices that guide us to optimal physical, mental, and emotional health.

We extend to you the opportunity to let us know how you are doing, and to find loving support on your compassionate journey of continual change and transformation. We encourage you to post on our blog times when you have seen an instance in your life or in the lives of others when love trumped fear. We ask you to consider offering kind support and thoughtful suggestions to others as we all discover what it means to love ourselves and others more deeply, and enter into lives of magnificent service to all. We invite you to find additional insights and to share your comments with our community at www.lovetrumpsfear.com. And, in the process, we all will continue to heal our hearts and transform our health, one day at a time.

ENDNOTES

Chapter 1

1. "The Bowl of Light," http://sovereigntyoflove.com/the-book/introduction-the-bowl-of-light.

2. Van Allsburg, Chris. *The Polar Express.* New York: Houghton Mifflin; 1st edition (October 28, 1985).

3. Peterson, Eugene, trans. *The Message: The Bible in Contemporary Language,* Genesis 27:1-40. NavPress, Feb. 2014.

4. Hay, Louise L. *You Can Heal Your Life.* Carlsbad, CA: Hay House, 1999, pp. 74-75.

Chapter 2

1. Reiss, Uzzi, MD, with Martin Zucker. *Natural Hormone Balance for Women: Look Younger, Feel Stronger, and Live Life with Exuberance.* Utria Books, January 2002.

2. Northrup, Christiane, MD. *The Wisdom of Menopause: Creating Physical and Emotional Health*

During the Change (Revised Edition). Bantam, January 2012.

3. Northrup, Christiane, MD. *Women's Bodies, Women's Wisdom: Creating Physical and Emotional Health and Healing* (Revised Edition). Bantam, June 2010.

4. Shoupe, Donna. "Individualizing hormone therapy to minimize risk: accurate assessment of risks and benefits." *Women's Health* (2011); 7(4): 475-85.

5. "NAMS Position Statement on Estrogen and Progestogen in Postmenopausal Women," 6/25/09, http://www.medscape.com/viewarticle/ 704910_print.

6. Newcomb, Polly A. et al. "Estrogen plus progestin use, microsatellite instability, and the risk of colorectal cancer in women." *Cancer Res* (2007 Aug 1); 67(15): 7534-7539.

7. Wroolie, Tonita E. "Differences in verbal memory performance in postmenopausal women receiving hormone therapy: 17β-estradiol versus conjugated equine estrogens." *Am J Geriatr Psychiatry* (2011 Sept); 19(9): 792-802.

8. Canonico M, Plu-Bureau G, Lowe GDO, Scarabin, PY. "Hormone replacement therapy and risk of venous thromboembolism in postmenopausal women: systematic review and meta-analysis." *BMJ* (2008 Mar 26); online first: 1-9.

9. LaCroix, Andrea et al. "Health outcomes after stopping conjugated equine estrogens among

postmenopausal women with prior hysterectomy: a randomized controlled trial." *JAMA* (April 6, 2011); 305(13): 1305-1313.

10. Holtorf, K. "The bioidentical hormone debate: are bioidentical hormones (estradiol, estriol, and progesterone) safer or more efficacious than commonly used synthetic versions in hormone replacement therapy? *Postgrad Med.* (2009 Jul); 121(4): 172.

11. Goodman, Michael P. "Are All Estrogens Created Equal? A Review of Oral vs. Transdermal Therapy." *Journal of Women's Health* (2012); 21(2): 161-169.

12. Brown, Richard P, Gerbarg, Patricia L, and Ramazanov, Zakir. "Rhodiola rosea: a Phytomedicinal Overview. *The Journal of the American Botanical Council* (2002); Issue 56: 40-52.

13. Weil, Andrew, MD. "Herbs," http:// www.drweil.com/drw/u/PAG00326/Herbs-Dr-Weil.html.

14. Gottfried, Sara, MD. *The Hormone Cure: Reclaim Balance, Sleep, and Sex Drive; Lose Weight; Feel Focused, Vital, and Energized Naturally with the Gottfried Protocol.* Scribner, March 2014.

15. Rankin, Lissa, MD. *Mind Over Medicine: Scientific Proof that You Can Heal Yourself.* Hay House, May 2013.

16. Erika Schwartz, MD. *The Hormone Solution: Naturally Alleviate Symptoms of Hormone Imbalance*

from Adolescence Through Menopause. Grand Central Publishing, April 2002.

17. Abraham Morgentaler, MD. *Testosterone For Life: Recharge Your Vitality, Sex Drive, Muscle Mass, and Overall Health.* McGraw Hill, November 2008.

18. Tan, Robert S., MD. *The Andropause Mystery: Unraveling Truths About the Male Menopause.* Amred Publishing, March 2009.

Chapter 3

1. LeWine, Howard, MD. Harvard Health Blog, http://www.health.harvard.edu/blog/hearts-fountain-of-youth-starts-flowing-early-201201274160.

2. Lipton, Bruce H., PhD. *The Biology of Belief: Unleashing the Power of Consciousness, Matter, & Miracles.* Hay House, November 2007.

3. Katz, David, MD, MPH. Web MD, http://www.webmd.com/diet/features/lose-weight-gain-tons-of-benefits.

4. Barnard, Neal D., MD. *21-Day Weight Loss Kickstart: Boost Metabolism, Lower Cholesterol, and Dramatically Improve Your Health.* Grand Central Life and Style, March 2013.

5. Patrick-Goudreau, Colleen. To learn more about Colleen's philosophy, go to www.joyfulvegan.com, or listen to her weekly podcast "Food for Thought."

Chapter 4

1. Brown, pp. 40-52.

2. Weil, "Rhodiola," http://www.drweil.com/drw/u/REM00033/Rhodiola-Dr-Weils-Herbal-Remedies.html.

3. "Vitamins and Supplements Lifestyle Guide, SAM-e," http://www.webmd.com/vitamins-and-supplements/lifestyle-guide-11/supplement-guide-sam-e.

4. Weil, "Herbs."

5. Weil, "Holy Basil to Combat Stress," http://www.drweil.com/drw/u/QAA346157/holy-basil-to-combat-stress.html.

6. Weekes, Claire, Dr. *Hope and Help for Your Nerves.* Signet, September 1990.

7. Weil, Andrew, MD. *Spontaneous Happiness.* Little, Brown, and Company, November 2011.

8. Amen, Daniel G., MD. *Healing Anxiety and Depression,* Berkley Trade, December 2004.

Chapter 5

1. Jelinek, George. *Overcoming Multiple Sclerosis: An Evidence-Based Guide to Recovery.* Allen & Unwin, 2009, pp. 138-41.

2. Ibid., pp. 297-298.

3. Orloff, Judith, MD. *The Ecstasy of Surrender: 12 Surprising Ways Letting Go Can Empower Your Life.* Harmony, 2014, p. 310.

4. Weil, "Herbs."

Chapter 6

1. Pert, Candace B., PhD. *Molecules of Emotion: The Science Behind Mind-Body Medicine.* Simon & Schuster, February 1999.

2. Amen, Daniel G., MD. *Change Your Brain, Change Your Life: The Breakthrough Program for Conquering Anxiety, Depression, Obsessiveness, Anger, and Impulsiveness.* Three Rivers Press, December 1998.

3. Benson, Herbert, MD and Miriam Z. Clipper. *The Relaxation Response.* Harper Torch, November 2000.

4. Chopra, Deepak, MD. *Perfect Health: The Complete Mind/Body Guide*, Revised and Updated Edition. Three Rivers Press, February 2001.

5. Dyer, Wayne W., PhD. *Change Your Thoughts, Change Your Life: Living the Wisdom of the Tao.* Hay House, January 2009.

6. Kabat-Zinn, Jon, Dr. *Full Catastrophe Living* (Revised Edition): Using the Wisdom of Your Body and Mind to Face Stress, Pain, and Illness. Bantam, September 2013.

7. Northrup, *Women's Bodies.*

8. Schultz, Mona Lisa, MD, PhD. *Awakening Intuition: Using Your Mind-Body Network for Insight and Healing.* Harmony, April 1999.

9. Carlson, Richard, PhD. *Don't Sweat the Small Stuff... and It's All Small Stuff.* Hyperion, January 1997.

10. Hay, *You Can Heal Your Life.*

11. Amen, *Change Your Brain, Change Your Life,* pp. 60-66.

Chapter 7

1. Naparstek, Belleruth. "Healthjourneys," www.healthjourneys.com.

2. www.chopra.com.

3. Kabat-Zinn, Jon, Dr. "Mindful Living Programs," www.mindfullivingprograms.com/whatMBSR.php.

4. www.osho.com.

5. Weil, Andrew MD. "Missing Out on Meditation," http://www.drweil.com/drw/u/id/QAA326653.

6. Brown, Dallas. "Three Reasons to Meditate," http://www.chopra.com/ccl/3-reasons-to-meditate.

7. Jelinek, p. 195.

Chapter 8

1. "Chinese Parable: Good Luck, Bad Luck" told by Karl Tong, https://www.youtube.com/watch?v=URo_vYEL5W8.

2. The poem *If* by Rudyard Kipling is available at http://www.poetryfondation.org/poem/175772.

3. Williamson, Marianne. "A Year of Daily Wisdom: A Perpetual Flip Calendar to Use Year After Year," June 19 entry. Hay House, 2005.

4. Beckwith, Rickie Byars. "We Let the Love Wash Over Us. https://www.youtube.com/watch?v=ImW01SvAyxo.

5. "Stranger Than Fiction," http://www.amazon.com/Stranger-Than-Fiction-Will-Ferrell/dp/B000LXH0AE.

INDEX

PUBLICATIONS AND ENDORSEMENTS

Love Trumps Fear: 8 Medical Insights to Heal Your Heart and Transform Your Life is Dr. Bilhartz's first book length publication. Her previous professional publications include:

Bilhartz, TD and Bilhartz, PA. "Occupation as a Risk Factor for Hypertensive Disorders of Pregnancy." *Journal of Women's Health* (Jan 25, 2013); 22(2): 1-9

Stocks J, Glazer C, Levin J, Huff S, Saito R, and Bilhartz P. "Obliterative Bronchiolitis in 2 Coffee-Processing Facility Workers – Texas, 2008-2012." *MMWR* (April 26, 2013); 62(16):305-307.

Bilhartz, TD, Bilhartz, PA, Bilhartz, TN, Bilhartz, RD. "Making Use of a Natural Stress Test: Pregnancy and Cardiovascular Risk." *Journal of Women's Health* (2011 May); 20(5):695-701.

Bilhartz, TD and Bilhartz, PA. "Navigating the Perfect Storm: Confronting the Epidemic of Hypertensive Disorders in Pregnancy." *Journal of Medical Humanities & Social Studies of Science and Technology* (2010 December); 2(2), ISSN 1852-4680.

Bilhartz, PA. Editorial, "Response to 'Transfusion-Associated Babesiosis: Shouldn't We Be Ticked Off?'" *Annals of Internal Medicine* (September 18, 2011).

The following excerpts are taken from reviews of *Love Trumps Fear* by notable medical and nutritional experts in the field:

"*Love Trumps Fear* is a beautifully organized and written blueprint for compassionately creating optimal health and healing. And getting right to the heart of the issue—whether it's anxiety, weight gain, panic, or a tumor! No matter what has happened to you or no matter what you're currently dealing with, *Love Trumps Fear* has the medicine you need to truly heal."

- Christiane Northrup, M.D., ob/gyn physician and author of the *New York Times* bestsellers: *Women's Bodies, Women's Wisdom* and *The Wisdom of Menopause*

-

"A book that balances mind, body and spirit to create total health."

-Judith Orloff, M.D., best-selling author of The *Ecstasy of Surrender*

"If you get to know Patty Bilhartz M.D., you will find that she is truly an amazing person! She has gone through so much in her personal life and shares from her heart. In *Love Trumps Fear* she speaks as both a patient and an accomplished physician. This is a good read, the first step for healing for many illnesses including endocrinological, psychological and neurological ones."

- Robert Tan M.D., author of *The Andropause Mystery: Unraveling Truths about the Male Menopause*

"*Love Trumps Fear* beautifully illustrates the benefits of a compassionate lifestyle. An enlightened read for those who want to live a life of joy!"

- Colleen Patrick-Goudreau, best-selling author of *The Joy of Vegan Baking* and *The 30-Day Vegan Challenge*

ABOUT GREEN
PUBLISHING HOUSE

MISSION

Green Publishing House is a Limited Liability Company dedicated to the production and global distribution of scholarly, peer-reviewed, academic books and high quality general interest trade books. Green Publishing House partners with numerous distributors to deliver valued books across multiple platforms (digital and print) at competitive costs.

The central mission of Green Publishing House is to deliver high quality digital textbooks and trade books to readers at low prices. Going digital is not only environmentally responsible and less expensive to readers, but it also offers our clients the opportunity to receive up-to-date scholarly resources on a moment's notice from millions of locations worldwide.

Although the number of digital readers is growing every year, because everyone may not have access to the internet and eBook readers, and because some individuals, book reviewers, and libraries may prefer hard copy texts, the company also offers print copies of its books. To remain loyal to its central mission, however, the company encourages the purchase of digital versions of its books, and cheerfully donates a portion of the revenue it receives from its print copy sales to educational and charitable institutions.

FOR AUTHORS

Green Publishing House currently is expanding its lists in the following areas:

- Health and Medicine
- History and Biography
- Religion and Spirituality
- Sports and Popular Culture

If you are an author working in one of these areas and would like to learn more about publishing opportunities with Green Publishing House, we invite you to visit the "For Authors" page at our website: www.GreenPublishingHouse.com.

www.ingramcontent.com/pod-product-compliance
Lightning Source LLC
Chambersburg PA
CBHW060902280326
41934CB00007B/1156